World report on road traffic injury prevention

Edited by
Margie Peden, Richard Scurfield,
David Sleet, Dinesh Mohan,
Adnan A. Hyder, Eva Jarawan
and Colin Mathers

World Health Organization

D1218678

WHO Library Cataloguing-in-Publication Data

World report on road traffic injury prevention / edited by Margie Peden … [et al.].
    1.Accidents, Traffic – prevention and control 2.Accidents, Traffic – trends
    3.Safety 4.Risk factors 5.Public policy 6.World health. I.Peden, Margie

    ISBN 92 4 156260 9   (NLM classification: WA 275)

© **World Health Organization 2004**

All rights reserved. Publications of the World Health Organization can be obtained from Marketing and Dissemination, World Health Organization, 20 Avenue Appia, 1211 Geneva 27, Switzerland (tel: +41 22 791 2476; fax: +41 22 791 4857; e-mail: bookorders@who.int). Requests for permission to reproduce or translate WHO publications – whether for sale or for noncommercial distribution – should be addressed to Publications, at the above address (fax: +41 22 791 4806; e-mail: permissions@who.int).

The designations employed and the presentation of the material in this publication do not imply the expression of any opinion whatsoever on the part of the World Health Organization concerning the legal status of any country, territory, city or area or of its authorities, or concerning the delimitation of its frontiers or boundaries. Dotted lines on maps represent approximate border lines for which there may not yet be full agreement.

The mention of specific companies or of certain manufacturers' products does not imply that they are endorsed or recommended by the World Health Organization in preference to others of a similar nature that are not mentioned. Errors and omissions excepted, the names of proprietary products are distinguished by initial capital letters.

The World Health Organization does not warrant that the information contained in this publication is complete and correct and shall not be liable for any damages incurred as a result of its use.

The named editors alone are responsible for the views expressed in this publication.

Designed by minimum graphics.
Cover by Tushita Graphic Vision.
Typeset and printed in Switzerland.

Contents

Foreword

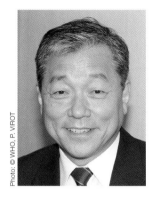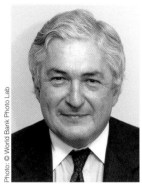

Every day thousands of people are killed and injured on our roads. Men, women or children walking, biking or riding to school or work, playing in the streets or setting out on long trips, will never return home, leaving behind shattered families and communities. Millions of people each year will spend long weeks in hospital after severe crashes and many will never be able to live, work or play as they used to do. Current efforts to address road safety are minimal in comparison to this growing human suffering.

The World Health Organization and the World Bank have jointly produced this *World report on road traffic injury prevention*. Its purpose is to present a comprehensive overview of what is known about the magnitude, risk factors and impact of road traffic injuries, and about ways to prevent and lessen the impact of road crashes. The document is the outcome of a collaborative effort by institutions and individuals. Coordinated by the World Health Organization and the World Bank, over 100 experts, from all continents and different sectors – including transport, engineering, health, police, education and civil society – have worked to produce the report.

Road traffic injuries are a growing public health issue, disproportionately affecting vulnerable groups of road users, including the poor. More than half the people killed in traffic crashes are young adults aged between 15 and 44 years – often the breadwinners in a family. Furthermore, road traffic injuries cost low-income and middle-income countries between 1% and 2% of their gross national product – more than the total development aid received by these countries.

But road traffic crashes and injuries are preventable. In high-income countries, an established set of interventions have contributed to significant reductions in the incidence and impact of road traffic injuries. These include the enforcement of legislation to control speed and alcohol consumption, mandating the use of seat-belts and crash helmets, and the safer design and use of roads and vehicles. Reduction in road traffic injuries can contribute to the attainment of the Millennium Development Goals that aim to halve extreme poverty and significantly reduce child mortality.

Road traffic injury prevention must be incorporated into a broad range of activities, such as the development and management of road infrastructure, the provision of safer vehicles, law enforcement, mobility planning, the provision of health and hospital services, child welfare services, and urban and environmental planning. The health sector is an important partner in this process. Its roles are to strengthen the evidence base, provide appropriate pre-hospital and hospital care and rehabilitation, conduct advocacy, and contribute to the implementation and evaluation of interventions.

The time to act is now. Road safety is no accident. It requires strong political will and concerted, sustained efforts across a range of sectors. Acting now will save lives. We urge governments, as well as other sectors of society, to embrace and implement the key recommendations of this report.

LEE Jong-wook
Director-General
World Health Organization

James D Wolfensohn
President
World Bank Group

Preface

Over 3000 Kenyans are killed on our roads every year, most of them between the ages of 15 and 44 years. The cost to our economy from these accidents is in excess of US$ 50 million exclusive of the actual loss of life. The Kenyan government appreciates that road traffic injuries are a major public health problem amenable to prevention.

In 2003, the newly formed Government of the National Alliance Rainbow Coalition, took up the road safety challenge. It is focusing on specific measures to curtail the prevalent disregard of traffic regulations and mandating speed limiters in public service vehicles.

Along with the above measures the Government has also launched a six-month Road Safety Campaign and declared war on corruption, which contributes directly and indirectly to the country's unacceptably high levels of road traffic accidents.

I urge all nations to implement the recommendations of the *World report on road traffic injury prevention* as a guide to promoting road safety in their countries. With this tool in hand, I look forward to working with my colleagues in health, transport, education and other sectors to more fully address this major public health problem.

Mwai Kibaki, President, Republic of Kenya

In 2004, World Health Day, organized by the World Health Organization, will for the first time be devoted to Road Safety. Every year, according to the statistics, 1.2 million people are known to die in road accidents worldwide. Millions of others sustain injuries, with some suffering permanent disabilities. No country is spared this toll in lives and suffering, which strikes the young particularly. Enormous human potential is being destroyed, with also grave social and economic consequences. Road safety is thus a major public health issue throughout the world.

World Health Day will be officially launched in Paris on 7 April 2004. France is honoured. It sees this as recognition of the major efforts made by the French population as a whole, which mobilized to reduce the death and destruction it faces on the roads. These efforts will only achieve results if they are supported by a genuine refusal to accept road accidents fatalistically and a determination to overcome all-too-frequent indifference and resignation. The mobilization of the French Government and the relevant institutions, particularly civic organizations, together with a strong accident prevention and monitoring policy, reduced traffic fatalities in France by 20%, from 7242 in 2002 to 5732 in 2003. Much remains to be done, but one thing is already clear: it is by changing mentalities that we will, together, manage to win this collective and individual struggle for life.

Jacques Chirac, President, France

Globally deaths and injuries resulting from road traffic crashes are a major and growing public health problem. Viet Nam has not been spared. In the year 2002, the global mortality rate due to traffic accidents was 19 per 100 000 population while in Viet Nam the figure was 27 per 100 000 population. Road traffic collisions on the nation's roads claim five times more lives now than they did ten years ago. In 2003 a total of 20 774 incidents were reported, leading to 12 864 deaths, 20 704 injuries and thousands of billions of Viet Nam Dong in costs.

A main contributor to road crashes in Viet Nam is the rapid increase in the number of vehicles, particularly motorcycles, which increase by 10% every year. Nearly half of the motorcycle riders are not licensed, and three quarters don't comply with traffic laws. Also, the development of roads and other transport infrastructure has not been able to keep pace with rapid economic growth.

To reduce deaths and injuries, protect property and contribute to sustainable development, the Government of Viet Nam established the National Committee on Traffic Safety in 1995. In 2001 the Government promulgated the National Policy on Accidents and Injury Prevention with the target of reducing traffic deaths to 9 per 10 000 vehicles. Government initiatives to reduce traffic accidents include issuing new traffic regulations and strengthening traffic law enforcement. In 2003, the number of traffic accidents was reduced by 27.2% over the previous year, while the deaths and injury rates declined by 8.1% and 34.8% respectively.

The Government of Viet Nam will implement more stringent measures to reduce road traffic injuries through health promotion campaigns, consolidation of the injury surveillance system, and mobilization of various sectors at all levels and the whole society. The Government of Viet Nam welcomes the World Health Organization/World Bank *World report on road traffic injury prevention,* and is committed to implementing its recommendations to the fullest extent possible.

H.E. Mr Phan Van Khai, Prime Minister, Socialist Republic of Viet Nam

In Thailand road accidents are considered one of the top three public health problems in the country. Despite the Government's best efforts, there are sadly over 13 000 deaths and more than one million injuries each year as the result of road accidents, with several hundred thousand people disabled. An overwhelming majority of the deaths and injuries involve motorcyclists, cyclists and pedestrians.

The Royal Thai Government regards this problem to be of great urgency and has accorded it high priority in the national agenda. We are also aware of the fact that effective and sustainable prevention of such injuries can only be achieved through concerted multisectoral collaboration.

To deal with this crucial problem, the Government has established a Road Safety Operations Centre encompassing the different sectors of the country and comprising the government agencies concerned, nongovernmental organizations and civil society. The Centre has undertaken many injury prevention initiatives, including a "Don't Drink and Drive" campaign as well as a campaign to encourage motorcyclists to wear safety helmets and to engage in safe driving practices. In this regard, we are well aware that such a campaign must involve not only public relations and education but also stringent law enforcement measures.

The problem of road traffic injuries is indeed a highly serious one, but it is also a problem that can be dealt with and prevented through concerted action among all the parties concerned. Through the leadership and strong commitment of the Government, we are confident that we will be successful in our efforts and we hope that others will be as well.

Thaksin Shinawatra, Prime Minister, Thailand

We are pleased that the Sultanate of Oman, with other countries, has brought up the issue of road safety to the United Nations General Assembly and played a major role in raising global awareness to the growing impact of deadly road traffic injuries, especially in the developing world.

The magnitude of the problem, encouraged the United Nations General Assembly to adopt a special resolution (No 58/9), and the World Health Organization to declare the year 2004 as the year of road safety.

In taking these two important steps, both organizations started the world battle against trauma caused by road accidents, and we hope that all sectors of our societies will cooperate to achieve this noble humanitarian objective.

The world report on road traffic injury prevention is no doubt a compelling reading document. We congratulate the World Health Organization and the World Bank for producing such a magnificent presentation.

Qaboos bin Said, Sultan of Oman

Land transportation systems have become a crucial component of modernity. By speeding up communications and the transport of goods and people, they have generated a revolution in contemporary economic and social relations.

However, incorporating new technology has not come about without cost: environmental contamination, urban stress and deteriorating air quality are directly linked to modern land transport systems. Above all, transportation is increasingly associated with the rise in road accidents and premature deaths, as well as physical and psychological handicaps. Losses are not limited to reduced worker productivity and trauma affecting a victim's private life. Equally significant are the rising costs in health services and the added burden on public finances.

In developing countries the situation is made worse by rapid and unplanned urbanization. The absence of adequate infrastructure in our cities, together with the lack of a legal regulatory framework, make the exponential rise in the number of road accidents all the more worrying. The statistics show that in Brazil, 30 000 people die every year in road accidents. Of these, 44% are between 20 and 39 years of age, and 82% are men.

As in other Latin American countries, there is a growing awareness in Brazil as to the urgency of reversing this trend. The Brazilian Government, through the Ministry of Cities, has put considerable effort into developing and implementing road security, education campaigns and programmes that emphasize citizen involvement. As part of this endeavour Brazil recently adopted a new road traffic code that has brought down the annual number of road deaths by about 5000. This is a welcome development that should spur us to even further progress. The challenges are enormous and must not be side stepped. This is why road security will remain a priority for my Government.

The publication of this report is therefore extremely timely. The data and analysis that it brings to light will provide valuable material for a systematic and in-depth debate on an issue that affects the health of all. Of even greater significance is the fact that the report will help reinforce our conviction that adequate preventive measures can have a dramatic impact. The decision to dedicate the 2004 World Health Day to *Road Safety* points to the international community's determination to ensure that modern means of land transportation are increasingly a force for development and the well-being of our peoples.

Luis Inácio Lula da Silva, President, Federative Republic of Brazil

Contributors

Editorial guidance
Editorial Committee
Margie Peden, Richard Scurfield, David Sleet, Dinesh Mohan, Adnan A. Hyder, Eva Jarawan, Colin Mathers.

Executive Editor
Margie Peden.

Advisory Committee
Eric Bernes, Suzanne Binder, John Flora, Etienne Krug, Maryvonne Plessis-Fraissard, Jeffrey Runge, David Silcock, Eduardo Vasconcellos, David Ward.

Contributors to individual chapters
Chapter 1. The fundamentals
Chair of Technical Committee: Ian Johnston.
Members of Technical Committee: Julie Abraham, Meleckidzedeck Khayesi, Vinand Nantulya, Claes Tingvall.
Writers: Jeanne Breen with contributions from Angela Seay.
Boxes: Brian White (Box 1.1); Hugo Acero (Box 1.2); Adnan A. Hyder (Box 1.3); Claes Tingvall (Box 1.4); Jeanne Breen (Box 1.5).

Chapter 2. The global impact
Chair of Technical Committee: Robyn Norton.
Members of Technical Committee: Abdulbari Bener, Maureen Cropper, Gopalkrishna Gururaj, El-Sayed Hesham, Goff Jacobs, Kara McGee, Chamaiparn Santikarn, Wang Zheng-gu.
Writers: Angela Seay with contributions from Andrew Downing, Meleckidzedeck Khayesi, Kara McGee, Margie Peden.
Boxes: Vinand Nantulya, Michael Reich (Box 2.1); David Sleet (Box 2.2); Ian Scott (Box 2.3); Liisa Hakamies-Blomqvist (Box 2.4); Chamaiparn Santikarn (Box 2.5); Lasse Hantula, Pekka Sulander, Veli-Pekka Kallberg (Box 2.6).

Chapter 3. Risk factors
Chair of Technical Committee: Murray MacKay.
Members of Technical Committee: Peter Elsenaar, Abdul Ghaffar, Martha Hijar, Veli-Pekka Kallberg, Michael Linnan, Wilson Odero, Mark Stevenson, Elaine Wodzin.
Writer: Jeanne Breen.
Boxes: Joelle Sleiman (Box 3.1); Anesh Sukhai, Ashley van Niekerk (Box 3.2).

Chapter 4. Interventions

Chair of Technical Committee: Ian Roberts.

Members of Technical Committee: Anthony Bliss, Jeanne Breen, Marcel Haegi, Todd Litman, Jack McLean, Ted Miller, Charles Mock, Nicole Muhlrad, Francesca Racioppi, Ralf Risser, Geetam Tiwari, Radin Umar, Maria Vegega, Dean Wilkerson.

Writer: Jeanne Breen with contributions from David Sleet, Angela Seay.

Boxes: Ruth Shults, Dorothy Begg, Daniel Mayhew, Herb Simpson (Box 4.1); Jeanne Breen (Box 4.2); Frances Afukaar (Box 4.3); Jeanne Breen (Box 4.4); Mark Stevenson (Box 4.5); Olivier Duperrex (Box 4.6).

Chapter 5. Conclusions and recommendations

Chair of Technical Committee: Fred Wegman.

Members of Technical committee: Andrew Downing, Ben Eijbergen, Frank Haight, Olive Kobusingye, Brian O'Neill, Ian Scott, David Silcock, Rochelle Sobel, Eduardo Vazquez-Vela, Rick Waxweiler.

Writer: Margie Peden.

Boxes: Ian Roberts (Box 5.1); Roy Antonio Rojas Vargas (Box 5.2).

Statistical Annex

Maureen Cropper, Kara McGee, Amy Li, Elizabeth Kopits, Margie Peden, Niels Tomijima.

Peer reviewers

Julie Abraham, Frances Afukaar, Noble Appiah, David Bishai, Christine Branche, Walter Buylaert, Witaya Chadbunchachai, Ann Dellinger, Jane Dion, Claude Dussault, Rune Elvik, Brendan Halleman, Alejandro Herrera, Ivan Hodac, Regina Karega, Arthur Kellermann, Martin Koubek, Jess Kraus, Larry Lonero, Mary McKay, Kate McMahon, Rose McMurray, Isabelle Mélèse, Heiner Monheim, Frederick Nafukho, Krishnan Rajam, Elihu Richter, Mark Rosenberg, Hans van Holst, Mathew Varghese, Maria Vegega, Philip Wambugu, Rick Waxweiler, Geert Wets, Paul White, John Whitelegg, Moira Winslow, Ingrida Zurlyte.

Additional contributors

Adielah Anderson, Abdulbari Bener, Anthony Bliss, Witaya Chadbunchachai, Carlos Dora, Marcel Dubouloz, Nelmarie du Toit, Randy Elder, Bill Frith, Sue Goldstein, Philip Graitcer, Marcel Haegi, Narelle Haworth, Christina Inclan, Arthur Kellerman, Rajam Krishnan, Risto Kumala, Larry Lonero, Stein Lundebye, Rick Martinez, Margaret McIntyre, Frederico Montero, Jim Nichols, Stephanie Pratt, Junaid Razzak, Donald Redelmeier, Richard Sattin, Ruth Shults, Rochelle Sobel, Grant Strachan, Leif Svanstrom, Tamitza Toroyan, Sebastian Van As, Hugh Waters, Wu Yuan.

Regional consultants

WHO African Region / Eastern Mediterranean Region

Hussain Abouzaid, Abdallah Assaedi, Sussan Bassiri, Abdhulbari Bener, Abdul Ghaffar, Mehdi Ghoya, Alaa Hamed, El-Sayed Hesham, Syed Jaffar Hussain, Mojahed Jameel, Tsegazeab Kebede, Meleckidzedeck Khayesi, Olive Kobusingye, Charlotte Ndiaye, Wilson Odero, Ian Roberts, Emmanuel Yoro Gouali.

WHO Region of the Americas

Julie Abraham, Anthony Bliss, Bryna Brennan, Alberto Concha-Eastman, Martha Hijar, Eva Jarawan, Larry Lonero, Kara McGee, Margie Peden, Deysi Rodriguez, Roy Antonio Rojas Vargas, Mark Rosenberg, Angela Seay, Richard Scurfield, Anamaria Testa Tambellini, Maria Vegega, Elisabeth Ward, Rick Waxweiler.

WHO South-East Asia Region / Western Pacific Region

Shanthi Ameratunga, Anthony Bliss, Li Dan, Sitaleki Finau, Gopalakrishna Gururaj, Ian Johnston, Rajam Krishnan, Robyn Norton, Munkdorjiin Otgon, Margie Peden, Chamaiparn Santikarn, Ian Scott, Gyanendra Sharma, Mark Stevenson, Madan Upadhyaya.

WHO European Region

Anthony Bliss, Piero Borgia, Jeanne Breen, Andrew Downing, Brigitte Lantz, Lucianne Licari, Margie Peden, Francesca Racioppi, Ian Roberts, Angela Seay, Laura Sminkey, Agis Tsouros, Jaroslav Volf, Ingrida Zurlyte.

Acknowledgements

The World Health Organization and the World Bank would like to acknowledge the members of the committees, regional consultation participants, peer reviewers, advisers and consultants, from over 40 countries, whose dedication, support and expertise made this report possible.

The World Health Organization, the World Bank and the Editorial Committee would like to pay a special tribute to Patricia Waller, who passed away on 15 August 2003. She was a member of the technical committee for chapter 1 but sadly became too ill to participate. Her many contributions to the promotion of road safety in the context of public health are acknowledged. She was a friend and mentor to many.

The report also benefited from the contributions of a number of other people. In particular, acknowledgement is made to Jeanne Breen and Angela Seay for writing the report under very tight time constraints, to Tony Kahane for editing the final text, to Stuart Adams for writing the summary and David Breuer for editing the summary. Thanks are also due to the following: Caroline Allsopp and Marie Fitzsimmons, for their invaluable editorial support; Anthony Bliss for technical support on transport-related matters; Meleckidzedeck Khayesi and Tamitza Toroyan, for assistance with the day-to-day management and coordination of the project; Kara McGee and Niels Tomijima, for statistical assistance; Susan Kaplan and Ann Morgan, for proofreading; Tushita Bosonet and Sue Hobbs, for graphic design and layout; Liza Furnival for indexing; Keith Wynn for production; Desiree Kogevinas, Laura Sminkey and Sabine van Tuyll van Serooskerken, for communications; Wouter Nachtergaele for assistance with references; Kevin Nantulya for research assistance; and Simone Colairo, Pascale Lanvers-Casasola, Angela Swetloff-Coff, for administrative support.

The World Health Organization also wishes to thank the following for their generous financial support for the development and publication of the report: the Arab Gulf Programme for United Nations Development Organizations (AGFUND); the FIA Foundation; the Flemish Government; the Global Forum for Health Research; the Swedish International Development Agency; the United Kingdom Department for Transport, Road Safety Division; the United States National Highway Traffic Safety Administration and the United States Centers for Disease Control and Prevention.

Introduction

Road traffic injuries constitute a major public health and development crisis, and are predicted to increase if road safety is not addressed adequately by Member States. The World Health Organization (WHO) has been concerned with this issue for over four decades. As early as 1962, a WHO report discussed the nature and dynamics of the problem (*1*). In 1974, the World Health Assembly adopted Resolution WHA27.59, declaring road traffic accidents a major public health issue and calling for Member States to address the problem (*2*). For the past two decades, the World Bank has encouraged its borrowers to include road safety components within most of their highway and urban transport projects.

Over the last three years, both organizations have intensified their work in road traffic injury prevention. This was reflected in the establishment in March 2000 of WHO's Department of Injuries and Violence Prevention, the development and implementation of a five-year WHO strategy for road traffic injury prevention, and greater financial and human support for road traffic injury prevention activities around the world (*3*). Recently, WHO dedicated World Health Day for 2004 to Road Safety. Within the World Bank, an interdisciplinary task force was established to ensure that this important issue was regarded as a major public health issue and tackled jointly by transport and public health specialists.

Among other international organizations, the United Nations Economic Commission for Europe, the United Nations Development Fund and the United Nations Children's Fund, have all stepped up their road safety activities over the past decade. In early 2003, the United Nations adopted Resolution (A/RES/57/309) on the global road safety crisis (*4*), followed by a report of the Secretary-General on the same topic to the 58th session of the United Nations General Assembly later that year (*5*). In November 2003, a further Resolution (A/RES/58/9) was passed by the United Nations, calling for a plenary meeting of the United Nations General Assembly on 14 April 2004. The purpose of the plenary meeting would be to increase awareness of the magnitude of the road injury problem, and to discuss the implementation of the *World report on road traffic injury prevention* at the United Nations General Assembly (*6*).

This joint WHO/World Bank report on road traffic injury prevention is an important part of the response to the world's road safety crisis. It is directed at international, regional and national policy-makers, international agencies and key professionals in public health, transport, engineering, education and other sectors, and aims to stimulate action for road safety. It sets out universal principles rather than a "blue print" for worldwide application, recognizing fully the need to identify local needs and the adaptation of "best practices" accordingly. A summary of the report is also available at http://www.who.int/violence_injury_prevention.

Aims of the report

The central theme of this report is the burden of road traffic injuries and the urgent need for governments and other key players to increase and sustain action to prevent road traffic injury.

The report's goals are:
— to raise awareness about the magnitude, risk factors and impacts of road traffic collisions globally;
— to draw attention to the preventability of the problem and present known intervention strategies;

— to call for a coordinated approach across a range of sectors to address the problem.

The specific objectives of the report are:

— to describe the burden, intensity, pattern and impacts of road traffic injuries at global, regional and national levels;

— to examine the key determinants and risk factors;

— to discuss interventions and strategies that can be employed to address the problem;

— to make recommendations for action at local, national and international levels.

The report elaborates on these objectives in five core chapters, described below.

The fundamentals

Chapter 1 gives an account of how the approach to road safety has developed over the years. It explains that the steep rise in road injury globally forecast over the next two decades is not inevitable if appropriate action is taken. The chapter argues the case for a multisectoral, systems-based approach to road injury prevention and mitigation.

The global impact

In Chapter 2, the defining characteristics and scale of the road traffic injury problem for different road users are laid out. The key issue of data collection is discussed and the impact of road traffic casualties on individuals, families and society in general is examined.

Risk factors

Chapter 3 describes the key risk factors and determinants for road crashes and road traffic injuries.

Interventions

Chapter 4 looks at possible interventions and discusses their effectiveness, cost and public acceptability, where such evidence is available.

Conclusions and recommendations

The final chapter draws conclusions and sets out the report's key recommendations for all those concerned with the safety of road traffic systems.

How the report was developed

Over 100 international professionals from the sectors of health, transport, engineering, law enforcement and education – among others – as well as the private sector and nongovernmental organizations, were involved in the development of this report. A small Editorial Committee coordinated this process. The outline for each chapter was developed by a Technical Committee with experts from all over the world. Two main writers wrote the various chapters of the report, after which the chapters were further refined by a stylistic editor. An Advisory Committee provided guidance to the Editorial Committee at the different stages of the report's production.

A series of consultations was held in the WHO regional offices with local experts and government officials to review the chapter outlines and make suggestions for the report's key recommendations. A meeting of the Technical Committee at WHO headquarters in Geneva further developed the work of the regional consultations on Chapter 5 – the chapter with the recommendations.

Prior to editing, each chapter was peer-reviewed by scientists and experts from around the world. These reviewers were asked to comment not only on the scientific content, but also on the relevance of each chapter within their local culture.

What happens after the report?

It is hoped that the launch of this report will mark the beginning of a long process of improving road safety. If it is to be effective, the report should stimulate discussion at local, national and international levels, and the recommendations should serve to bring about greatly increased actions on road traffic injury prevention around the world.

References

1. Norman LG. *Road traffic accidents: epidemiology, control, and prevention.* Geneva, World Health Organization, 1962.
2. Resolution WHA27.59. Prevention of road traffic accidents. In: *Twenty-seventh World Health Assembly, Geneva, 7–23 May 1974.* Geneva, World Health Organization, 1974 (http://www.who.int/violence_injury_prevention/media/en/171.pdf, accessed 17 November 2003).
3. Peden M et al. *A 5-year WHO strategy for road traffic injury prevention.* Geneva, World Health Organization, 2001 (http://whqlibdoc.who.int/hq/2001/WHO_NMH_VIP_01.03.pdf, accessed 30 October 2003).
4. *United Nations General Assembly resolution 57/309 on global road safety crisis (22 May 2003).* New York, NY, United Nations (http://www.unece.org/trans/roadsafe/docs/GA_R_57-309e.pdf, accessed 30 October 2003).
5. United Nations General Assembly. *Global road safety crisis: report of the Secretary-General (7 August 2003).* New York, NY, United Nations (A/58/228) (http://www.who.int/world-health-day/2004/infomaterials/en/un_en.pdf, accessed 30 October 2003).
6. *United Nations General Assembly resolution A/RES/58/9 on global road safety crisis (19 November 2003).* New York, NY, United Nations (http://ods-dds-ny.un.org/doc/UNDOC/GEN/N03/453/45/PDF/N0345345.pdf?Open Element, accessed 30 December 2003).

CHAPTER 1

The fundamentals

Introduction

Road traffic injuries are a major but neglected global public health problem, requiring concerted efforts for effective and sustainable prevention. Of all the systems that people have to deal with on a daily basis, road transport is the most complex and the most dangerous. Worldwide, the number of people killed in road traffic crashes each year is estimated at almost 1.2 million, while the number injured could be as high as 50 million – the combined population of five of the world's large cities. The tragedy behind these figures regularly attracts less media attention than other, less frequent but more unusual types of tragedy.

What is worse, without increased efforts and new initiatives, the total number of road traffic deaths worldwide and injuries is forecast to rise by some 65% between 2000 and 2020 (1, 2), and in low-income and middle-income countries deaths are expected to increase by as much as 80%. The majority of such deaths are currently among "vulnerable road users" – pedestrians, pedal cyclists and motorcyclists. In high-income countries, deaths among car occupants continue to be predominant, but the risks per capita that vulnerable road users face are high.

This is the first major report on road injury prevention jointly issued by the World Health Organization (WHO) and the World Bank, and underscores the concern that the two bodies share about the detrimental impact of an unsafe road transport system on public health and global development. It is the contention of the report, first, that the level of road deaths and injuries is unacceptable, and second, that it is to a large extent avoidable.

There is thus an urgent need to recognize the worsening situation in road deaths and injuries and to take appropriate action. Road traffic injury prevention and mitigation should be given the same attention and scale of resources that is currently paid to other prominent health issues if increasing human loss and injury on the roads, with their devastating human impact and large economic cost to society, are to be averted.

The report has three main aims:
- To create a greater level of awareness, commitment and informed decision-making at all levels – including among governments, professional sectors and international agencies – so that strategies scientifically proven to be effective in preventing road injuries can be implemented. Any effective response to the global challenge of reducing traffic casualties will necessarily require a large mobilization of effort by all those concerned, at the international, national and local levels.
- To provide a sound justification for the change in thinking that has taken place in recent years, especially where significant research has been undertaken, about the nature of the road traffic injury problem and what constitutes successful prevention. The perception that it is the price to be paid for achieving mobility and economic development, needs to be replaced by a more holistic ideology that places the emphasis on the total system of road traffic.
- To help strengthen institutions and create effective partnerships to deliver safer road traffic systems. Such partnerships should exist horizontally between different sectors of government and vertically between different levels of government, as well as between governments and nongovernmental organizations. At governmental level this means establishing a close collaboration between the sectors of transport, public health, finance, the judiciary and others concerned.

The report is thus principally aimed at policy-makers and key professionals in all sectors and at all levels, with an objective to provide a strategic framework for action. Universal principles are set out, rather than a single action plan with worldwide applicability. This is because local conditions must always be taken into account, so that best practices proven elsewhere can be refined and adapted into relevant and successful local interventions.

A public health concern

Road deaths, disability and injury

Every day around the world, almost 16 000 people die from all types of injuries. Injuries represent 12% of the global burden of disease, the third most important cause of overall mortality and the main cause of death among 1–40-year-olds (3). The category of injuries worldwide is dominated by those incurred in road crashes. According to WHO data, deaths from road traffic injuries account for around 25% of all deaths from injury (4).

Estimates of the annual number of road deaths vary, as a result of the limitations of injury data collection and analysis, problems of underreporting and differences in interpretation. The figure ranges from around 750 000 (5) (probably an underestimate, since it is made on the basis of 1998 data) to 1 183 492 annually – representing over 3000 lives lost daily (see Statistical Annex, Table A.2).

Around 85% of all global road deaths, 90% of the disability-adjusted life years lost due to crashes, and 96% of all children killed worldwide as a result of road traffic injuries occur in low-income and middle-income countries. Over 50% of deaths are among young adults in the age range of 15–44 years (6). Among both children aged 5–14 years, and young people aged 15–29 years, road traffic injuries are the second-leading cause of death worldwide (see Table 1.1).

TABLE 1.1

Leading causes of deaths by age group, world, 2002

Rank	0–4 years	5–14 years	15–29 years	30–44 years	45–59 years	≥60 years	All ages
1	Lower respiratory infections 1 890 008	Childhood cluster diseases 219 434	HIV/AIDS 707 277	HIV/AIDS 1 178 856	Ischaemic heart disease 1 043 978	Ischaemic heart disease 5 812 863	Ischaemic heart disease 7 153 056
2	Diarrhoeal diseases 1 577 891	Road traffic injuries 130 835	Road traffic injuries 302 208	Tuberculosis 390 004	Cerebrovascular disease 623 099	Cerebrovascular disease 4 685 722	Cerebrovascular disease 5 489 591
3	Low birth weight 1 149 168	Lower respiratory infections 127 782	Self-inflicted injuries 251 806	Road traffic injuries 285 457	Tuberculosis 400 704	Chronic obstructive pulmonary diseases 2 396 739	Lower respiratory infections 3 764 415
4	Malaria 1 098 446	HIV/AIDS 108 090	Tuberculosis 245 818	Ischaemic heart disease 231 340	HIV/AIDS 390 267	Lower respiratory infections 1 395 611	HIV/AIDS 2 818 762
5	Childhood cluster diseases 1 046 177	Drowning 86 327	Interpersonal violence 216 169	Self-inflicted injuries 230 490	Chronic obstructive pulmonary diseases 309 726	Trachea, bronchus, lung cancers 927 889	Chronic obstructive pulmonary diseases 2 743 509
6	Birth asphyxia and birth trauma 729 066	Malaria 76 257	Lower respiratory infections 92 522	Interpersonal violence 165 796	Trachea, bronchus, lung cancers 261 860	Diabetes mellitus 749 977	Diarrhoeal diseases 1 766 447
7	HIV/AIDS 370 706	Tropical cluster diseases 35 454	Fires 90 845	Cerebrovascular disease 124 417	Cirrhosis of the liver 250 208	Hypertensive heart disease 732 262	Childhood-cluster diseases 1 359 548
8	Congenital heart anomalies 223 569	Fires 33 046	Drowning 87 499	Cirrhosis of the liver 100 101	Road traffic injuries 221 776	Stomach cancer 605 395	Tuberculosis 1 605 063
9	Protein–energy malnutrition 138 197	Tuberculosis 32 762	War 71 680	Lower respiratory infections 98 232	Self-inflicted injuries 189 215	Tuberculosis 495 199	Trachea, bronchus, lung cancers 1 238 417
10	STDs excluding HIV 67 871	Protein–energy malnutrition 30 763	Hypertensive disorders 61 711	Poisonings 81 930	Stomach cancer 185 188	Colon and rectum cancers 476 902	Malaria 1 221 432
11	Meningitis 64 255	Meningitis 30 694	Maternal haemorrhage 56 233	Fires 67 511	Liver cancer 180 117	Nephritis and nephrosis 440 708	Road traffic injuries 1 183 492
12	Drowning 57 287	Leukaemia 21 097	Ischaemic heart disease 53 870	Maternal haemorrhage 63 191	Diabetes mellitus 175 423	Alzheimer and other dementias 382 339	Low birth weight 1 149 172
13	Road traffic injuries 49 736	Falls 20 084	Poisoning 52 956	War 61 018	Lower respiratory infections 160 259	Liver cancer 367 503	Diabetes mellitus 982 175
14	Endocrine disorders 42 619	Violence 18 551	Childhood cluster diseases 48 101	Drowning 56 744	Breast cancer 147 489	Cirrhosis of the liver 366 417	Hypertensive heart disease 903 612
15	Tuberculosis 40 574	Poisonings 18 529	Abortion 43 782	Liver cancer 55 486	Hypertensive heart disease 129 634	Oesophagus cancer 318 112	Self-inflicted injuries 874 955

Source: WHO Global Burden of Disease project, 2002, Version 1 (see Statistical Annex).

In low-income countries and regions – in Africa, Asia, the Caribbean and Latin America – the majority of road deaths are among pedestrians, passengers, cyclists, users of motorized two-wheelers, and occupants of buses and minibuses (*7, 8*). The leading casualties in most high-income countries, on the other hand, are among the occupants of cars.

However, when it comes to comparative fatality rates (deaths for any measure of exposure) for all users in the traffic system, these regional differences disappear. Nearly everywhere, the risk of dying in a road crash is far higher for vulnerable road users – pedestrians, cyclists and motorcyclists – than for car occupants (*8, 9*).

The road traffic death toll represents only the "tip of the iceberg" of the total waste of human and societal resources from road injuries. WHO estimates that, worldwide, between 20 million and 50 million people are injured or disabled each year in road traffic crashes (the reason for the wide range of this estimate being the considerable, known underreporting of casualties) (*10*).

Using epidemiological evidence from national studies, a conservative estimate can be obtained of the ratios between road deaths, injuries requiring hospital treatment, and minor injuries, as being 1:15:70 in most countries (*11–18*).

In many low-income and middle-income countries, the burden of traffic-related injuries is such that they represent between 30% and 86% of all trauma admissions (*19, 20*).

While a decrease in deaths due to road traffic crashes of some 30% is forecast in high-income countries, current and projected trends in low-income and middle-income countries foreshadow a huge escalation in global road crash mortality between 2000 and 2020. Furthermore, on current trends, by 2020, road crash injury is likely to be the third leading cause of disability-adjusted life years lost (see Table 1.2).

TABLE 1.2

Change in rank order of DALYs for the 10 leading causes of the global burden of disease

	1990		2020
Rank	Disease or injury	Rank	Disease or injury
1	Lower respiratory infections	1	Ischaemic heart disease
2	Diarrhoeal diseases	2	Unipolar major depression
3	Perinatal conditions	3	Road traffic injuries
4	Unipolar major depression	4	Cerebrovascular disease
5	Ischaemic heart disease	5	Chronic obstructive pulmonary disease
6	Cerebrovascular disease	6	Lower respiratory infections
7	Tuberculosis	7	Tuberculosis
8	Measles	8	War
9	Road traffic injuries	9	Diarrhoeal diseases
10	Congenital abnormalities	10	HIV

DALY: Disability-adjusted life year. A health-gap measure that combines information on the number of years lost from premature death with the loss of health from disability.
Source: reference *2*.

The social and economic costs of road traffic injuries

In economic terms, the cost of road crash injuries is estimated at roughly 1% of gross national product (GNP) in low-income countries, 1.5% in middle-income countries and 2% in high-income countries (*5*).

The direct economic costs of global road crashes have been estimated at US$ 518 billion, with the costs in low-income countries – estimated at US$ 65 billion – exceeding the total annual amount received in development assistance (*5*). Furthermore, the costs estimated for low-income and middle-income countries are probably significant underestimates. Using more comprehensive data and measurement techniques, the estimated annual costs (both direct and indirect) of road crash injury in European Union (EU) countries alone, which contribute 5% to the global death toll, exceed €180 billion (US$ 207 billion) (*9, 21*). For the United States of America, the human capital costs of road traffic crashes in 2000 were estimated at US$ 230 billion (*22*). If comparable estimates were made of the direct and indirect economic costs of road crashes in low-income and middle-income countries, the total economic cost globally of road crashes would be likely to exceed the current estimate of US$ 518 billion.

Road crashes not only place a heavy burden on national and regional economies but also on households (see Box 1.1). In Kenya, for example, more than 75% of road traffic casualties are among economically productive young adults (*23*).

Despite the large social and economic costs, though, there has been a relatively small amount of investment in road safety research and development, compared with other types of health loss (see Table 1.3).

There exist, however, well-tested, cost-effective and publicly-acceptable solutions to the problem. Funding for interventions, though, even in many countries most active in road safety – all of whom have targets for further reductions in casualties – has been scarce (*25–28*).

In short, current road safety efforts fail to match the severity of the problem. Road travel brings society benefits, but the price society is paying for it is very high.

BOX 1.1

The human tragedies behind road crash statistics

On a spring weekend in 2000, in the rural English setting of Suffolk, Ruth, 22 years old and her brother Paul, 20, joined their parents to celebrate their 25th wedding anniversary. After the family celebrations, on the Sunday evening, Paul went to a film, driven by a friend in his amateurly-repaired and rebuilt old Fiat Uno.

At midnight they heard the heavy knocking of a policeman, who announced that there had been a car crash and asked the shocked parents to attend the local hospital. The prognosis was terrible. Paul had suffered massive brain injury and was not expected to live. Strangely, he did not look so bad – many scratches and bruises, deep glass cuts to his left cheek, and broken fingers and femur – but the brain scan told a far worse story.

Paul was transferred to intensive care and, within hours, to the regional Neurosciences Critical Care Unit. Mercifully, they had a bed and knew how to provide the best care. However, his life hung by a thread. He had suffered severe injuries to his brain and lungs. The doctors kept Paul in a coma until he had stabilized. When he was allowed to come round, though, the family's worst fears were confirmed as the doctors talked about nerves severed from the brain stem.

Paul survived and now, over three years later, continues to progress, but painfully slowly, from a minimally-responsive, vegetative state. He still cannot walk or talk or write, so communication with him is very difficult. But he can now smile, and show pleasure or frustration. He can swallow and eat and, with the coordination in his right hand improving and with prompting, he can sometimes help himself to eat. He remains doubly-incontinent.

After a few months in a general hospital, Paul had six months of rehabilitation therapy and is now in a high-dependency home, 50 km from his parents. Additional therapy, support workers and equipment are paid for from interim compensation claims against the driver's insurance. Without these funds, and the tireless lobbying and much other work by his parents, his sister and others, Paul would not have progressed as far as he has.

Mum and Dad go to see Paul once a week, often timing the visit to coincide with discussions with doctors, managers or therapists. They bring Paul home most Saturdays and once a month overnight. Dad can only work three days a week now because of the load of duties related to Paul. Their house has been adapted to accommodate the wheelchair and provide for Paul's care needs.

The family has learnt to cope with the stress caused by the memory of the crash and its consequences. However, their trust and their attitude of "it won't happen to me or my close ones" has disappeared. Instead, there is agonized concern about road safety, the attitudes of drivers and the injustices of the legal system.

In this case, the young driver had driven so fast that, trying to take a corner, he caught the kerb, crossed the road, climbed a low bank and crashed the rear of the car into a tree. Paul was in the back and took the brunt of the impact. The back of the car broke off, due to the poor-quality "renovation" job on the rusted vehicle, which should never have been allowed to pass the compulsory annual vehicle test (the "MOT" test).

The system failed Paul's family by doing nothing about the dishonest MOT pass, and by bringing only a minor driving charge against the driver, with the offence of excess speed – and not of ruining Paul's life. On top of their suffering, Paul's parents have had to live with the injustices of the law, which they feel does not deal properly with crashes such as those of Paul, and pays inadequate attention to serious injury.

There can be a very fine dividing line between death and injury. For many months, the family grieved over the loss of Paul, who had before him all the hopes of a bright and promising young man – hopes that have long vanished.

TABLE 1.3

Estimated global research and development
funding for selected topics

Disease or injury	US$ millions	1990 DALYs ranking	2020 DALYs ranking
HIV/AIDS	919–985	2	10
Malaria	60	8	—
Diarrhoeal diseases	32	4	9
Road traffic crashes	24–33	9	3
Tuberculosis	19–33	—	7

DALYs: disability-adjusted life years.
Source: reference 24.

Changing fundamental perceptions

A key purpose of this report is to communicate current knowledge and thinking about road injury prevention to a wider audience involved in managing road safety. Since the last major WHO world report on road safety issued over 40 years ago (29), there has been a major change in the perception, understanding and practice of road injury prevention – a shift of paradigms – among traffic safety professionals around the world.

Figure 1.1 sets out the guiding principles of this paradigm. Some governments, some organizations, and some individuals will more easily and readily than others take on board their implications. The principles involved will not all be adopted at once but will take time to become firmly established, even in those countries where road safety is energetically pursued.

The following sections provide examples of how this new way of perceiving and dealing with road traffic safety is already affecting capacity building and policy. Also discussed are the types of measures found to be successful and the starting points for institutional and programme development. Chapter 4 examines further some of the programmes and interventions for road traffic safety that are suitable for local adoption and adaptation.

The predictability and preventability of road crash injury

One reason for the historical neglect of "injury" in public health is the traditional view of accidents and injuries as random events that happen to others (6, 30). Such events are looked upon as an inevitable outcome of road transport.

While the risk of a crash is relatively low for most individual journeys, people travel many times each day, every week and every year. The sum of these small risks is considerable. The term "accident", which is widely used, can give the impression, probably unintended, of inevitability and unpredictability – an event that cannot be managed. This document prefers to use the term "crash" instead, to denote something that is an event, or series of events, amenable to rational analysis and remedial action.

Many highly-motorized countries, in response to rising road trauma levels during the 1960s and early 1970s, achieved large reductions in casualties through outcome-oriented and science-based approaches. This response was stimulated by campaigners including Ralph Nader in the United States (31), and given intellectual strength by scientists such as William Haddon Jr (32, 33).

FIGURE 1.1

The road safety paradigm shift

ROAD INJURY PREVENTION AND CONTROL – THE NEW UNDERSTANDING

■ Road crash injury is largely preventable and predictable; it is a human-made problem amenable to rational analysis and countermeasure

■ Road safety is a multisectoral issue and a public health issue – all sectors, including health, need to be fully engaged in responsibility, activity and advocacy for road crash injury prevention

■ Common driving errors and common pedestrian behaviour should not lead to death and serious injury – the traffic system should help users to cope with increasingly demanding conditions

■ The vulnerability of the human body should be a limiting design parameter for the traffic system and speed management is central

■ Road crash injury is a social equity issue – equal protection to all road users should be aimed for since non-motor vehicle users bear a disproportionate share of road injury and risk

■ Technology transfer from high-income to low-income countries needs to fit local conditions and should address research-based local needs

■ Local knowledge needs to inform the implementation of local solutions

Experience shows that with political will and a commitment to achieve effective safety management, a rapid and significant reduction in road injuries can be achieved. The efforts required, as will be outlined in this report, include (*25, 34*):
— a scientific approach to the topic;
— the provision, careful analysis and interpretation of good data;
— the setting-up of targets and plans;
— the creation of national and regional research capacity;
— institutional cooperation across sectors.

The need for good data and a scientific approach

Road traffic injury prevention is a highly politicized issue. Most people have their own opinions on what could make the roads safer. Anecdotal information and its reporting by the media all too often allow issues to be understood as major traffic safety problems requiring priority action, which in turn puts pressure on policy-makers to respond. Policy decisions for effective road injury prevention need to be based on data and objective information, not on anecdotal evidence.

First, data on the incidence and types of crashes are needed. After that, a detailed understanding of the circumstances that lead to crashes is required to guide safety policy. Furthermore, knowledge of how injuries are caused and of what type they are is a valuable instrument for identifying interventions and for monitoring the effectiveness of interventions.

In many low-income and middle-income countries, systematic efforts to collect road traffic data are not well developed and underreporting of deaths and serious injuries is common. The health sector has an important responsibility to ensure that the necessary data systems are established and that data on the main injury problems and on the effectiveness of interventions are communicated to a wider audience.

Only by systematic and data-led management of the leading road injury problems will significant reductions in exposure to crash risk and in the severity of crashes be achieved.

Road safety as a public health issue

Traditionally, road traffic safety has been assumed to be the responsibility of the transport sector, with the main focus within this sector limited to building infrastructure and managing traffic growth.

Road safety agencies and research institutes

With the sharp increases in motorization in the 1960s in many developed countries, traffic safety agencies were often set up, usually located within a government's transport department. Often, though, there was little coordination between these bodies and other government departments with responsibilities relating to road safety, either nationally or locally. In some cases, for example, vehicle safety standards had been developed by departments dealing with trade and industry, while traffic law enforcement was dealt with at the local or regional level, controlled by the justice department. In general, the public health sector was slow to become involved (*34–38*).

A second development was the creation of national technical and scientific support bodies on road traffic, in which road safety decision-making formed a part. Examples included the Swedish National Road and Traffic Research Institute created in 1971, the United Kingdom Road Research Laboratory (now TRL Ltd), and the Accident Research Units in Adelaide and Sydney, Australia, as well as the Australian Road Research Board. In the United States, such research units were embedded within the national traffic safety agency so as to feed more directly into policy-making. Formal advisory bodies, such as the National Transportation Safety Board and the Transportation Research Board (part of the United States National Academy of Sciences), were also set up to provide independent advice and guidance.

The combination of new, dedicated institutes on road safety and greater scientific research has in many cases produced major changes in thinking about traffic safety and in interventions (*34*). However, at the same time, there is often a real conflict between the aims of traffic safety lobbies and those of campaigners for increased mobility or for environmental concerns. In such cases, the lobby for mobility has frequently been the dominant one. In the long term, increases in mobility, without the corresponding necessary increases in safety levels, will have a negative effect on public health (*39*).

The focus on mobility has meant investment in constructing and maintaining infrastructure – that is, cars and roads – for private and commercial motorized transport, to the relative neglect of public transport and of the safety of non-motorized road users such as pedestrians and cyclists. This has placed a heavy burden on the health sector.

Road crash injuries are indeed a major public health issue, and not just an offshoot of vehicular mobility. The health sector would greatly benefit from better road injury prevention in terms of fewer hospital admissions and a reduced severity of injuries. It would also be to the health sector's gain if – with safer conditions on the roads guaranteed for pedestrians and cyclists – more people were to adopt the healthier lifestyle of walking or cycling, without fearing for their safety.

The public health approach

The public health approach to road traffic injury prevention is based on science. The approach draws on knowledge from medicine, biomechanics, epidemiology, sociology, behavioural science, criminology, education, economics, engineering and other disciplines.

While the health sector is only one of many bodies involved in road safety – and usually not even the leading one – it nonetheless has important roles to play (see Figure 1.2). These include:

- discovering, through injury surveillance and surveys, as much as possible about all aspects of road crash injury – by systematically collecting data on the magnitude, scope, characteristics and consequences of road traffic crashes;
- researching the *causes* of traffic crashes and injuries, and in doing so trying to determine:
  — causes and correlates of road crash injury,
  — factors that increase or decrease risk,
  — factors that might be modifiable through interventions;
- exploring ways to prevent and reduce the severity of injuries in road crashes – by designing, implementing, monitoring and evaluating appropriate interventions;
- helping to implement, across a range of settings, interventions that appear promising, especially in the area of human behaviour, disseminating information on the outcomes, and evaluating the cost-effectiveness of these programmes;
- working to persuade policy-makers and decision-makers of the necessity to address injuries in general as a major issue, and of the importance of adopting improved approaches to road traffic safety;
- translating effective science-based information into policies and practices that protect pedestrians, cyclists and the occupants of vehicles;
- promoting capacity building in all these areas, particularly in the gathering of information and in research.

FIGURE 1.2

Road traffic injury as a public health problem

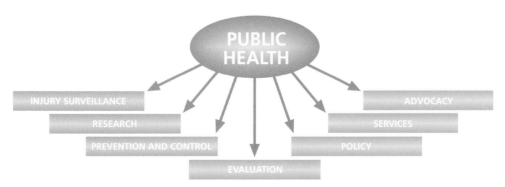

Cross-sectoral collaboration is essential here, and this is something the public health sector is in a good position to promote.

Road safety as a social equity issue

Studies show that motor vehicle crashes have a disproportionate impact on the poor and vulnerable in society. These are also the people with usually little influence over policy decisions (*40, 41*). Even in high-income countries, poor children are at greater risk than children from more prosperous families (*41–43*).

Poorer people comprise the majority of casualties and lack ongoing support in the event of long-term injury. Lower socioeconomic groups have limited access to post-crash emergency health care (*44*). In addition, in many developing countries, the costs of prolonged medical care, the loss of the family breadwinner, the cost of a funeral, and the loss of income due to disability can push families into poverty (*45*). In Mexico, the second commonest cause of children being orphaned is traffic crashes (*45*).

In developing countries, the population groups exposed to the highest risks of injury and death from road crashes – for example, pedestrians and users of motorized two-wheelers – are from lower socioeconomic groups (*40, 46*). They face a greater likelihood of injury, since affordable transport poses higher risks in these places than private car use.

A large proportion of the road crash victims in low-income and middle-income countries are pedestrians and cyclists. They benefit the least from policies designed for motorized travel, but bear a disproportionate share of the disadvantages of motorization in terms of injury, pollution and the separation of communities.

In high-income countries, the risks associated with walking, cycling and motorcycling remain very high in relation to those of car travel – the principal focus of urban and rural highway provision since motorization levels rose sharply in the 1960s (*47, 48*).

In many countries, the absence of a voice for the most vulnerable groups has meant that the safety of pedestrians and cyclists is often disregarded in favour of motorized travel.

Equal protection for all road users should be a guiding rule, to avoid an unfair burden of injury and death for poorer people and vulnerable road users (*40, 49*). This issue of equity is a central one for reducing the global burden of road crash death and injury.

Systems that accommodate human error

The traditional view in road safety has been that when crashes occur, they are usually the sole responsibility of individual road users, despite the fact that other factors beyond their control may have come into play, such as the poor design of roads or vehicles. It is still widely held today that since human error is a factor in some 90% of road crashes, the leading response should be to persuade road users to adopt "error-free" behaviour. According to this policy, information and publicity should form the backbone of road traffic injury prevention, rather than being one element of a much more comprehensive programme (*50, 51*).

Human error on the roads does not always lead to disastrous consequences. Error by a road user, though, may indeed trigger a crash, but not necessarily be its underlying cause. In addition, human behaviour is governed not only by individual knowledge and skills, but also by the environment in which the behaviour takes place (*52*). Indirect influences, such as the design and layout of the road, the nature of the vehicle, and traffic laws and their enforcement – or lack of enforcement – affect behaviour in important ways. For this reason, the use of information and publicity on their own is generally unsuccessful in reducing road traffic collisions (*26, 34, 35, 53*).

Error is part of the human condition. Aspects of human behaviour in the context of road traffic safety can certainly be altered. Nonetheless, errors can also be effectively reduced by changing the immediate environment, rather than focusing solely on changing the human condition (*54*).

In the field of road safety, it has proved difficult to overcome the traditional overreliance on single approaches (*26, 34, 39, 55, 56*). Road safety policymakers in north-western Europe are increasingly acknowledging, though, that the road traffic system needs to ensure, through its design and operation, that it does not lead to significant public health loss (*57, 58*).

None of the above contradicts the strict need for individuals to comply with key safety rules and to avoid dangerous situations (*52, 55*). However, as the Swedish Committee of Inquiry into Road Traffic Responsibility concluded (*59*):

> *In order to achieve a safe transport system, there must be a change in our views concerning responsibility, to the extent that system designers are given clearly defined responsibility for designing the road system on the basis of actual human capabilities, thereby preventing the occurrence of those cases of death and serious injury that are possible to predict and prevent.*

Systems that account for the vulnerability of the human body

The uncertainty of human behaviour in a complex traffic environment means that it is unrealistic to expect that all crashes can be prevented. However, if greater attention in designing the transport system were given to the tolerance of the human body to injury, there could be substantial benefits. It is certainly within the bounds of possibility to try to ensure that if crashes do occur, they do not, as a matter of course, lead to serious public health loss.

In the majority of serious and fatal crashes, injuries are caused because loads and accelerations, exceeding those the body can tolerate, are applied by some part of the car (*60*). Pedestrians, for example, incur a risk of about 80% of being killed at a collision speed of 50 kilometres/hour (km/h), as opposed to a 10% risk at speeds of 30 km/h. At speeds of over 30 km/h, motorists, pedestrians and cyclists increasingly make mistakes, the consequences of which are often fatal. The human tolerance to injury for a pedestrian hit by a car will be exceeded if the vehicle is travelling at over 30 km/h (*61*).

Most traffic systems, however, whether in developing or developed countries, go beyond these limits on a regular basis. Separating cars and pedestrians on the road by providing pavements is very often not done. Speed limits of 30 km/h in shared-space residential areas are commonly not implemented. Car and bus fronts, as generally designed, do not provide protection for pedestrians against injury at collision speeds of 30 km/h or greater.

For car occupants, wearing seat-belts in well-designed cars can provide protection to a maximum of 70 km/h in frontal impacts and 50 km/h in side impacts (*61*). Higher speeds could be tolerated if the interface between the road infrastructure and vehicle were to be well-designed and crash-protective – for example, by the provision of crash cushions on sharp ends of roadside barriers. However, most infrastructure and speed limits in existence today allow much higher speeds without the presence of crash-protective interfaces between vehicle and roadside objects, and without significant use of seat-belts. This is particularly the case in many low-income and middle-income countries.

In all regions of the world, to prevent road death and disabling injury, a traffic system better adapted to the physical vulnerabilities of its users needs to be created – with the use of more crash-protective vehicles and roadsides.

Technology transfer from high-income countries

Transport systems developed in high-income countries may not fit well with the safety needs of low-income and middle-income countries for a variety of reasons, including the differences in traffic mix (*50, 62, 63*).

In low-income countries, walking, cycling, motorcycling and use of public transport are the predominant transport modes. In North America and Europe, there are between two and three people per car. In China and India, on the other hand, there are 280 and 220 people per car, respectively (*64*), and while it is predicted that car ownership will increase in these countries, it will still remain low in terms of cars per capita for another 20–30 years (*49*).

In developing countries, roads often carry a wide range of users – from heavy good vehicles to bicycles and pedestrians without any separation. Among the pedestrians, the most vulnerable are children and older people. The motorized traffic on these roads is capable of high acceleration and speed, both key factors in the causes of road crash injury.

Technology transfer, therefore, needs to be appropriate for the mix of different vehicle types and the patterns of road use in a particular place (*65*).

Road safety in countries that are in the process of becoming motorized is further hindered by the perception that current levels of walking, cycling and motorcycling are temporary. Such a view may have arisen through imported expertise from developed countries as much as from domestic sources (*66*). This tends to lead to models of infrastructure from developed countries being adopted to cater to the *longer-term* transport needs. However, in most low-income countries, safety should be promoted within *existing* conditions, and these include: low per capita incomes, the presence of mixed traffic, a low capacity for capital intensive infrastructure, and a different situation as regards law enforcement (*50*).

In high-income settings, new strategies and programmes for traffic injury prevention generally require considerable analysis and planning before implementation. In developing countries, though, because of the scarcity of resources, the priority should be the import and adaptation of proven and promising methods from developed nations, and a pooling of information as to their effectiveness in the imported settings among other low-income countries (*67*).

The new model

In all parts of the world, whatever the level of motorization, there is a need to improve the safety of the traffic system for all its users, and to reduce current inequalities in the risk of incurring road crash injuries.

To achieve this, advances in road safety will require an approach that includes various key elements absent from previous efforts. This will entail policy-makers, decision-makers, professionals and practitioners recognizing that the traffic injury problem is an urgent one, but one for which solutions are already largely known. It will require that road safety strategies be integrated with other

strategic, and sometimes competing goals, such as those relating to the environment and to accessibility and mobility.

A key factor in tackling the growing road traffic injury burden is the creation of institutional capacity across a range of interlinking sectors, backed by both strong political commitment and adequate and sustainable resources.

A systems approach

An essential tool for effective road crash injury prevention is the adoption of a *systems approach* (*68*) to:

— identify problems;
— formulate strategy;
— set targets;
— monitor performance.

Road safety efforts must be evidence-based, fully costed, properly resourced and sustainable.

In the United States some 30 years ago, William Haddon Jr inspired safety professionals when he talked about road transport as an ill-designed, "man-machine" system needing comprehensive systemic treatment. He defined three phases of the time sequence of a crash event – pre-crash, crash and post-crash – as well as the epidemiological triad of human, machine and environment that can interact during each phase of a crash. The resulting nine-cell Haddon Matrix models a dynamic system, with each cell of the matrix allowing opportunities for intervention to reduce road crash injury (*32*) (see Figure 1.3).

This work led to substantial advances in the understanding of the behavioural, road-related and vehicle-related factors that affect the number and severity of casualties in road traffic. The "systems" approach seeks to identify and rectify the major sources of error or design weakness that contribute to fatal and severe injury crashes, as well as to mitigate the severity and consequences of injury.

Building on Haddon's insights, a wide range of strategies and techniques for casualty reduction have since been tested internationally, through scientific research and empirical observation. The strategies (discussed further in Chapter 4) include interventions:

FIGURE 1.3

The Haddon Matrix

PHASE		FACTORS		
		HUMAN	**VEHICLES AND EQUIPMENT**	**ENVIRONMENT**
Pre-crash	Crash prevention	Information Attitudes Impairment Police enforcement	Roadworthiness Lighting Braking Handling Speed management	Road design and road layout Speed limits Pedestrian facilities
Crash	Injury prevention during the crash	Use of restraints Impairment	Occupant restraints Other safety devices Crash-protective design	Crash-protective roadside objects
Post-crash	Life sustaining	First-aid skill Access to medics	Ease of access Fire risk	Rescue facilities Congestion

— to reduce exposure to risk;
— to prevent road traffic crashes from occurring;
— to reduce the severity of injury in the event of a crash;
— to reduce the consequences of injury through improved post-collision care.

This systemic approach to interventions is targeted and carried out within a broader system of managing safety.

Building capacity for systemic safety management is a long-term process that in high-income countries has developed over an extended period of motorization and the growth and reform of institutions. In low-income and middle-income countries, systemic safety management is generally weaker, and needs to be strengthened.

Evidence from North America, Australia and Europe shows that integrated strategic programmes produce a marked decline in road deaths and serious injuries (*34, 69, 70*). A recent review of countries with the lowest death rates – the Netherlands, Sweden and the United Kingdom – concluded that while it was accepted that there was scope for improvement, their progress had been due to continuing planned systemic improvements over recent decades aimed at vehicles, roads and users (*25*). Chapter 4 discusses the measures that have contributed to the relative successes of these programmes.

While progress has been made in many highly-motorized countries, the practical realization of the systems approach remains the most important challenge for road safety policy-makers and professionals.

At the same time, there are plenty of examples of the mistakes that highly-motorized nations have made in attempts to improve safety. If newly-motorizing nations could avoid such mistakes, a large proportion of road crash injuries could be avoided (*26, 56, 64*). Such mistakes include:
— the failure to adopt strategies or interventions based on evidence;
— expenditure on ineffective but easy policy options;
— a focus on the mobility of vehicle users at the expense of the safety of vulnerable road users;
— insufficient attention to the design of traffic systems and insufficient professional scrutiny of the detail of traffic safety policy.

The errors also included those of omission, as opportunities to prevent deaths and injuries by measures such as the design of better vehicles and less hazardous roadsides, and improving trauma care systems, were in many cases missed (*56*).

Developing institutional capacity

The development of traffic safety policy involves a wide range of participants representing a diverse group of interests (see Figure 1.4). In many countries, responsibilities for road safety are spread over different levels of government with policy being decided at local, national and international levels. In the United States, for example, responsibilities are split between the federal government and the individual states. In EU countries, much of the regulation affecting vehicle safety is initiated centrally in Brussels, Belgium.

FIGURE 1.4

The key organizations influencing policy development

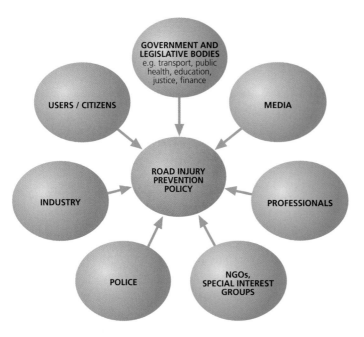

The construction of multisectoral institutional capacity, both in the governmental and non-governmental spheres, is a key to developing road safety, and can only be delivered by a national, political commitment (see Box 1.2). As Wesemann observes, there is sufficient evidence to show that free-market mechanisms are no substitute for government intervention when it comes to providing greater safety (71).

The role of government

Historically, in most highly-motorized countries, governmental responsibilities for traffic safety policy fall within the transport ministry or the police department. Other government departments such as those of justice, health, planning and education may also have responsibilities for key areas. In some instances, vehicle safety standards are handled by the department (or ministry) of industry.

Trinca et al. – in their historical analysis of how governments have dealt with road safety – conclude that in many cases the institutional arrangements for traffic safety have been fragmentary and lacking

a strong lead, and that road safety interests have been submerged by other competing interests (34).

The experience of several countries indicates that effective strategies for reducing traffic injury have a greater chance of being applied if there is a separate government agency with the power and the budget to plan and implement its programme (34). Examples of "stand-alone" traffic safety agencies are limited. However, in the 1960s, Sweden and the United States created traffic safety bodies, separate from the main transport departments, that oversaw the implementation, in a relatively short period of time, of a range of new road safety interventions.

The Swedish Road Safety Office (SRSO) was established in the late 1960s, with responsibility for road safety. Though it lacked significant powers or resources, the number of road deaths between 1970 and the mid-1980s was reduced each year. In 1993, the SRSO merged with the more powerful and better-resourced Swedish National Road Administration (SNRA), to which the ministry of transport and communications delegated full responsibility for road safety policy.

In the United States – against a background of sharply rising road casualties – the Highway Safety Act of 1970 created a traffic safety agency, the National Highway Traffic Safety Administration (NHTSA). NHTSA delivered the first set of vehicle safety standards and encouraged a new way of thinking about traffic safety strategy. The agency is responsible for reducing deaths, injuries and economic losses resulting from motor vehicle crashes. It aims to accomplish this by setting and enforcing safety performance standards for motor vehicles and motor vehicle equipment, and by providing grants to state and local governments to enable them to conduct effective local road safety programmes. NHTSA investigates safety defects in

BOX 1.2

Reducing traffic fatalities in Bogotá, Colombia

Over an eight-year period from 1995 to 2002, the Colombian capital, Bogotá, with a population of seven million, implemented a range of policies to reduce fatal and non-fatal injuries from external causes. As a result, the number of traffic-related deaths fell over the period by almost a half – from 1387 in 1995 to 697 in 2002.

The first measure was to set up a unified data system on violence and crime, designed by the Institute of Forensic Medicine and Science to gather data on deaths from violence, and in particular from traffic crashes. Using the statistics on road traffic crashes in Bogotá, the interagency Committee for Epidemiological Surveillance of Injuries from External Causes then produced a set of public policies aimed at reducing the number of accidents, improving mobility around the city and increasing the safety of road users.

Improving the performance and image of traffic police

The following year, 2000 traffic police who had failed to enforce traffic regulations and, in many cases, were guilty of corruption were replaced. Responsibility for regulating traffic and enforcing rules was transferred to the Metropolitan Police, which assigned more than 1000 officers and 500 auxiliaries to traffic duties. This police force now has a positive public image and concentrates exclusively on enforcing traffic discipline. Officers found acting corruptly are dismissed.

Since 1996, spot checks have been carried out for drunken driving. Drivers failing the test have their vehicles impounded and are fined around US$ 150. The media are closely involved with these checks, conducted on weekends at crash black spots. Speed cameras have also been set up on the city's main roads.

In 1998, the Colombian National University was commissioned to carry out research into traffic crashes. Based on their findings, further decisions to increase road safety were taken, including the construction of highways, pavements and pedestrian bridges. The study also identified individual behaviour that increased the risk of traffic injuries, and from this drew up civic education programmes on traffic safety.

Attempts to change behaviour

One of these programmes, launched by the city's mayor, was aimed at changing people's behaviour on the roads. Measures promoted included the wearing of safety belts and observing pedestrian crossings. While the Highway Code already included these rules and people were generally aware of them, most people had failed to observe them and the authorities had generally failed to enforce them.

In the programme, mime was used on numerous sites throughout Bogotá. The mime actors working for the programme used sign language to point out to drivers that they were not wearing seat-belts, or that they had failed to give way at pedestrian crossings. At first, drivers were simply warned and told to change their behaviour. If this failed, a traffic policeman stepped in and handed out a fine, to the applause of onlookers. Nowadays, over 95% of drivers have been found to observe these rules.

Converting space into pedestrian areas

Since 1996, radical steps have been taken to win back areas from street traders and seasonal vendors. Large public spaces that had been taken over by vendors or vehicles have been converted into pedestrian areas, with new pavements and pedestrian bridges constructed.

In addition to the traffic police, the administration employs some 500 guides in its Bogotá Mission programme – young people trained in traffic regulations, first aid, preventive safety measures and the detailed layout of the city. Their task is to encourage safe behaviour on public roads.

Mass transport system

A new mass transport system, known as the TransMilenio, has not only improved urban transport and mobility, but has also reduced the number of traffic injuries along its routes, with the construction of infrastructure to ensure the safety of pedestrians and other road users. Surrounding areas have also been improved with better lighting and other equipment to make the system safer, more user-friendly and more efficient.

motor vehicles, helps states and local communities deal with the threat posed by drunken drivers, promotes the use of safety belts, child safety seats and air bags, and provides consumer information on motor vehicle safety topics. NHTSA also conducts research on traffic safety and driver behaviour.

While giving responsibility for road safety to a stand-alone agency is likely to increase the priority given to road safety, strong political support and actions from other agencies are essential to bring about major changes (*72*). If the establishment of a stand-alone agency to coordinate activity is not possible, then an alternative is to strengthen the existing road safety unit, giving it greater powers within the government transport ministry (*34*).

The experience from a wide range of countries is that, whatever the organizational structure, it is important that the lead governmental organization for road safety should be clearly defined, with its specific responsibilities and coordinating roles set out (*66, 72*).

Parliamentary committees

Experience worldwide demonstrates that effective road safety policies can also arise out of the efforts of informed and committed members of parliament.

In the Australian state of New South Wales in the early 1980s, the Parliamentary Standing Committee on Road Safety was responsible for the introduction and full implementation of random breath testing, which led to a 20% reduction in deaths and – according to surveys – was supported by over 90% of people. Earlier, in the neighbouring state of Victoria, political action and a report by a parliamentary committee had led to the world's first legislation on the compulsory use of front seat-belts. The law in Victoria came into effect at the beginning of 1971; by the end of that year car occupant deaths had fallen by 18%, and by 1975 by 26% (*73*).

Joint groups comprising legislators and professionals can also make a valuable contribution. In the United Kingdom in the 1980s, for example, a cross-party coalition of members of parliament came together with concerned professionals and nongovernmental organizations to form the Parliamentary Advisory Council for Transport Safety (PACTS). The first success of the Council – which campaigned strongly for road safety policy to be based on evidence – was in having legislation passed for front seat-belt use. PACTS went on to argue for, and eventually see, the introduction of further measures, including speed humps and the use of rear seat-belts.

A sympathetic institutional climate needs to be built up where the mutual encouragement of road injury prevention professionals and policy-makers – both in the executive and the legislature – can provide a stimulus and effective response. It is important that legislative bodies provide both authorization and funding support to the relevant government agencies to carry out road safety initiatives.

Research

Rational decision-making in public policy is dependent on impartial research and information. Developing research capacity nationally is a central feature of the new model of road safety (*74, 75*) (see Box 1.3). Without research capacity, there exist few means to overcome misconceptions and prejudices about road crash injuries.

National and community research – as opposed to relying solely on international research – is important for identifying local problems and localized groups at increased risk of road injury. It also helps to ensure a cadre of national and local professionals who can use research findings to calculate the implications for policy and programmes. Furthermore, the national evaluation effort needs to be led by research professionals, since it is only through implementation and thorough evaluation that effective programmes evolve.

The independence of research and its separation from the executive function in developing public policy is necessary for ensuring quality and to protect the research body against short-term political pressures, but at the same time interaction between the two is essential (*34*).

There are many examples of the role of independent research effort carried out by universities and national research laboratories in developing national and international policy. The Transportation Research and Injury Prevention Programme at

BOX 1.3

Research capacity development

"Capacity development" is a broad concept covering the planning, development, implementation, evaluation and sustainability of a complex phenomenon. Efforts at capacity development in the field of health research have been conducted for several decades by international, bilateral and private organizations. Traditionally, such programmes provided funds to train scientists from the developing world in centres of excellence in developed countries. In the field of road traffic injury prevention, there are several types of initiative that can provide models for capacity development.

Network development at the institutional level allows for exchange of information, the sharing of experiences, and the fostering of collaborative projects and research studies. The WHO Collaborating Centres for Violence and Injury Prevention are one global example of this model. Another, at regional level, is the Injury Prevention Initiative for Africa.

Another model is to support schemes that allow scientists and professionals to exchange research ideas and findings, develop proposals, mentor younger researchers and carry out research directed at policy-making. The global Road Traffic Injury Research Network is an example of such a framework that focuses on researchers from low-income and middle-income countries.

A third model for capacity development is to strengthen university departments and research institutes in the developing world so as to generate a critical mass of appropriately trained professionals. The Indian Institute of Technology and Universiti Putra Malaysia are examples of centres with regular training programmes on road safety.

A fourth model is to strengthen career development pathways of trained professionals and to prevent their drain from low-income and middle-income countries. Both of these are important for attracting and retaining valuable human resources. Part of such a strategy includes establishing positions for road traffic injury prevention in appropriate ministries – such as those of health and transport – and finding incentives to encourage professionals in such posts to perform at a high level.

In recent years, there have been growing concerns about the impact of training programmes and attempts have been made to devise methods to evaluate them. Recent efforts initiated by the World Health Organization to assess national health research systems may provide useful tools to evaluate research capacity development as well.

the Institute of Technology in New Delhi, India, has contributed much to a better understanding of the road injury problems of vulnerable road users and to identifying possible interventions in low-income and middle-income countries – as has equally the Centre for Industrial and Scientific Research in South Africa.

There are Accident Research Units at universities in Adelaide and Melbourne, Australia; Loughborough, England; and Hanover, Germany. Among other work, these units gather crash injury information which feeds into the development of international vehicle safety standards. The former Transport Research Laboratory (now known as TRL Ltd) in the United Kingdom is known for its research and development work on European vehicle safety standards, which have helped reduce casualties among a large population. The Dutch

Institute for Road Safety Research (SWOV), which is independent of government, has made a significant contribution in the Netherlands (*58*). In the United States, academic institutes such as the North Carolina Highway Safety Research Center and the University of Michigan Transportation Research Institute, as well as government bodies such as NHTSA and the National Center for Injury Prevention and Control at the Centers for Disease Control and Prevention, have advanced research over several decades (*76*).

The involvement of industry

Industry shares responsibility for road injury prevention, in the design and use of its products and as an employer whose staff and transport services are often major road users. It also supports work on road traffic crashes and injuries. As one example, organizations funded by the insurance industry make a valuable contribution to road safety. Folksam in Sweden and the Insurance Institute for Highway Safety in the United States provide objective information about the crash performance of new cars and other safety issues. Data collection by the Finnish insurers' fund, which investigates every fatal crash occurring nationally and carries out safety studies, feeds directly into public information and policy.

Nongovernmental organizations

The nongovernmental sector can play a major role in road casualty reduction (*34*). Nongovernmental organizations (NGOs) serve road safety most effectively when they:

— publicize the true scale of the road injury problem;
— provide impartial information for use by policy-makers;
— identify and promote demonstrably-effective and publicly-acceptable solutions, with consideration as well of their cost;
— challenge ineffective policy options;
— form effective coalitions of organizations with a strong interest in casualty reduction;
— measure their success by their ability to influence the implementation of effective road casualty reduction measures (*77*).

An example of a road safety NGO is the Trauma Committee of the Royal Australasian College of Surgeons, set up in 1970. Its objectives include: establishing and maintaining the highest possible level of post-impact care for those injured in crashes; developing undergraduate and postgraduate training programmes; gathering and disseminating hard clinical data that can be used to identify traffic injury problems; actively promoting injury prevention measures; and supporting community awareness programmes (*34*).

In the 20 years since its inception, the advocacy efforts of Mothers Against Drunk Driving (MADD) have had remarkable success. The United States-based organization has witnessed the enactment of over 300 excess-alcohol laws between 1980 and 1986, the introduction of random sobriety check-

points, the elimination of plea bargaining for excess alcohol, mandatory prison sentences, and in many states, a minimum drinking age now set at 21 years.

The Brussels-based European Transport Safety Council (ETSC) provides an international example of successful coalition-building to achieve specific aims. Successful campaigns include a European Union-wide road fatality reduction target and new vehicle safety standard legislation. Since its inception in 1993, ETSC has pushed road safety to the centre of European Union transport policy-making and has had a remarkable influence on the work of the Road Safety and Technology Unit of the European Commission's Directorate-General for Energy and Transport and on the European Parliament's scrutiny of transport safety matters (*27*).

In developing countries, it is often difficult for organizations that want to campaign on road safety to obtain funding (*72*). However, there are several new victims' organizations and advocacy groups that have been set up in developing countries. Examples include: Asociación Familiares y Víctimas de Accidentes del Tránsito (Argentina) [Association of Families and Victims of Traffic Accidents]; Friends for Life (India); the Association for Safe International Road Travel (Kenya and Turkey); the Youth Association for Social Awareness (Lebanon); and Drive Alive (South Africa).

Achieving better performance

In the past 30 years, a new body of knowledge has been accumulated regarding effective road safety management and ways of measuring it. This section outlines examples of some of the most recent methods in traffic safety management. These include:

— management based on outcome or results, using objective information;
— targets to motivate professionals;
— acceptance of the idea of shared responsibility;
— partnerships between central and local government;
— partnerships involving other concerned bodies.

Shared responsibility

The approach for deciding how responsibility for safety on the roads should be shared is a pragmatic and ethical one, but with scientific foundations, particularly in the science of ergonomics. It recognizes that road deaths and serious injuries can be avoided by adopting a culture of safety involving all the key participants and by implementing important safety measures more widely and systematically (*55, 70*).

In the new paradigm, the principle of social responsibility involves the vehicle manufacturer providing crash protection inside and outside the vehicle. The vehicle uses a road system where conflict is minimized by design and energy transfer is controlled as far as possible. That system is then used by a community that complies with risk-avoiding behavioural norms created by education, legislation and enforcement (*55*).

In this model, designers and builders are an integral part of the systems approach to road safety (*55*). For the model to be effective, though, there must also be accountability and a means to measure performance objectively.

Two countries in particular have formally adopted the systems approach to road safety. Both Sweden and the Netherlands, as described in the following sections, have put into legislation models in which effective partnerships are the key method of delivering road safety plans, setting targets and introducing other safety performance indicators.

Safety performance indicators, related to crashes or injuries, provide a test for ensuring that actions are as effective as possible and represent the best use of public resources (*78*).

Sweden's "Vision Zero"

Vision Zero — so called because its ultimate goal is no fatalities or severe injuries through road traffic crashes — has public health as its underlying premise (*61*) (see Box 1.4). It is a road safety policy that puts the protection of the most vulnerable road users at its centre.

BOX 1.4

Vision Zero

Vision Zero is a traffic safety policy, developed in Sweden in the late 1990s and based on four elements: ethics, responsibility, a philosophy of safety, and creating mechanisms for change. The Swedish parliament voted in October 1997 to adopt this policy and since then several other countries have followed suit.

Ethics

Human life and health are paramount. According to Vision Zero, life and health should not be allowed in the long run to be traded off against the benefits of the road transport system, such as mobility. Mobility and accessibility are therefore functions of the inherent safety of the system, not vice versa as it is generally today.

Responsibility

Until recently, responsibility for crashes and injuries was placed principally on the individual road user. In Vision Zero, responsibility is *shared* between the providers of the system and the road users. The system designers and enforcers – such as those providing the road infrastructure, the car-making industry and the police – are responsible for the functioning of the system. At the same time, the road user is responsible for following basic rules, such as obeying speed limits and not driving while under the influence of alcohol. If the road users fail to follow such rules, the responsibility falls on the system designers to redesign the system, including rules and regulations.

Safety philosophy

In the past, the approach to road safety was generally to put the onus on the road user. In Vision Zero, this is replaced by an outlook that has been used with success in other fields. Its two premises are that:

    human beings make errors;

    there is a critical limit beyond which survival and recovery from an injury are not possible.

It is clear that a system that combines human beings with fast-moving, heavy machines will be very unstable.

BOX 1.4 (continued)

It is sufficient for a driver of a vehicle to lose control for just a fraction of a second for a human tragedy to occur. The road transport system should therefore be able to take account of human failings and absorb errors in such a way as to avoid deaths and serious injuries. Crashes and even minor injuries, on the other hand, need to be accepted. The important point is that the chain of events that leads to a death or disability must be broken, and in a way that is sustainable, so that over the longer time period loss of health is eliminated.

The limiting factor of this system is the human tolerance to mechanical force. The chain of events leading to a death or serious injury can be broken at any point. However, the *inherent* safety of the system – and that of the road user – is determined by people not being exposed to forces that go beyond human tolerance. The components of the road transport system – including road infrastructure, vehicles and systems of restraint – must therefore be designed in such a way that they are linked to each other. The amount of energy in the system must be kept below critical limits by ensuring that speed is restricted.

Driving mechanisms for change

To change the system involves following the first three elements of the policy. While society as a whole benefits from a safe road transport system in economic terms, Vision Zero relates to the citizen as an individual and his or her right to survive in a complex system. It is therefore the demand from the citizen for survival and health that is the main driving force. In Vision Zero, the providers and enforcers of the road transport system are responsible to citizens and must guarantee their safety in the long term. In so doing, they are necessarily required to cooperate with each other, for simply looking after their own individual components will not produce a safe system. At the same time, the road user has an obligation to comply with the basic rules of road safety.

In Sweden, the main measures undertaken to date include:
— setting safety performance goals for various parts of the road traffic system;
— a focus on vehicle crash protection, and support for the consumer information programme of the European New Car Assessment Programme (EuroNCAP);
— securing higher levels of seat-belt use and fitting smart, audible seat-belt reminders in new cars;
— installing crash-protective central barriers on single-carriageway rural roads;
— encouraging local authorities to implement 30 km/h zones;
— wider use of speed camera technology;
— an increase in the number of random breath tests;
— the promotion of safety as a competitive variable in road transport contracts.

While the Vision Zero does not say that the ambitions on road safety historically have been wrong, the actions that would have to be taken are partly different. The main differences probably can be found within how safety is being promoted; there are also some innovations that will come out as a result of the vision, especially in infrastructure and speed management.

A tool for all

Vision Zero is relevant to any country that aims to create a sustainable road transport system, and not just for the excessively ambitious or wealthy ones. Its basic principles can be applied to any type of road transport system, at any stage of development. Adopting Vision Zero means avoiding the usual costly process of trial and error, and using from the start a proven and effective method.

Vision Zero is a long-term strategy in which improvements are delivered in gradual increments, and where, over time, the responsibility for safety becomes shared by the designers and users of the road traffic system. The idea is that a system more tolerant of human limitations will lead eventually to a changed division of responsibility between the car industry, the health sector, road safety engineering and traffic planning (*61*).

According to the policy, if the inherent safety of the system cannot be changed, then the only radical way to reduce the road toll is to lower travel speeds. On the other hand, if a substantial reduction in vehicle speed is unacceptable, the alternative has to be investment to improve the inherent safety of the system, at a given level of desired mobility (*61*).

Investment in Sweden has been mainly directed at managing speed where there is a potential for conflict with other vehicles and providing better links between vehicle crash protection and the infrastructure. Other investments are being directed towards more protective roadsides and a greater separation of road users where speeds exceed 60–70 km/h. For pedestrian safety, the aim is to restrict vehicle speeds to 30 km/h where there are potential dangers between vehicles and pedestrians, or else physically to separate cars and pedestrians.

Setting an example, the Swedish National Road Administration has already instigated quality assurance for its own road transport operations and work-related road travel.

"Sustainable safety" in the Netherlands

Conceived by the Institute for Road Safety Research and the Dutch Ministry of Transport, and developed in cooperation with local authorities, a three-year programme on "sustainable safety" was launched in 1998 (see Box 1.5).

BOX 1.5

Sustainable safety: the example of the Netherlands

The increasing demands for mobility have unwanted and adverse consequences. Future generations, though, should not have to bear the heavy burden resulting from the demands of the present generation. The means exist now to reduce significantly the costly and largely avoidable tragedy of road casualties.

Aim
By 2010 in the Netherlands, road deaths should be reduced by at least 50% and injuries by 40%, compared with the 1986 baseline figures.

What is a safe and sustainable traffic system?
A road traffic system that is safe and sustainable will have the following features:

  its infrastructure will have been adapted to take into account human limitations, using proper road design;
  its vehicles will be equipped to make the task of driving easier and to provide a high standard of protection in crashes;
  its road users will be provided with adequate information and education and, where appropriate, will be deterred from undesirable or dangerous behaviour.

Strategic principles
There are three guiding principles in the strategy for a safe and sustainable road system. These are as follows:

  The road network should be reclassified according to *road function*, with a single and unambiguous function established for as many roads as possible. The three types of road function are:
  o the *flow function* – enabling high speeds for long-distance traffic, frequently also involving large volumes of traffic;
  o the *distributor function* – helping to distribute traffic to scattered destinations and serving regions and districts;
  o the *access function* – enabling direct access to properties alongside a road.
  Speed limits should be set according to road function.
  Using appropriate design, the function of roads, their layout and their use should be made compatible, by:
  o preventing the unintended use of roads;
  o preventing large discrepancies in speed, direction and volume at moderate and high speeds;
  o preventing confusion among road users by making the nature of roads more predictable.

Necessary actions
The actions needed to achieve the safe and sustainable road systems include:

  the creation of partnerships at national, regional and local levels to re-engineer the road network, with a greater emphasis on safety;
  a programme to be implemented in two phases, with a start-up period of two years, to reclassify the road network;
  a 30 km/h speed limit introduced as a general rule for all built-up areas, with powers given to local authorities to make exceptions.

As with the Swedish programme, the sustainable safety programme in the Netherlands takes, as its underlying premise, that "man is the measure of all things". Its key aim is to re-engineer and manage the road network so as to provide a safer system (*58*).

Speed management is a central theme. One of the goals is to convert as many urban roads as possible to a "residential" function, with a maximum speed limit of 30 km/h. Previous experience in the Netherlands with 30 km/h zones had shown that a casualty reduction of 22% could be achieved (*58*). Once it had been established that two thirds of the Dutch urban road network could be converted to 30 km/h zones, the programme – a joint operation between central and local government – reclassified the road network and by 2001 had converted as much as 50%

TABLE 1.4

Examples of current fatality reduction targets in use[a]

Country or area	Base year for target	Year in which target is to be realized	Target reduction in the number of road traffic fatalities
Australia	1997	2005	−10%
Austria	1998–2000	2010	−50%
Canada	1991–1996	2008–2010	−30%
Denmark	1998	2012	−40%
European Union	2000	2010	−50%
Finland	2000	2010	−37%
		2025	−75%
France	1997	2002	−50%
Greece	2000	2005	−20%
		2015	−40%
Ireland	1997	2002	−20%
Italy	1998–2000	2010	−40%
Malaysia	2001	2010	< 3 deaths/10 000 vehicles
Netherlands	1998	2010	−30%
New Zealand	1999	2010	−42%
Poland	1997–1999	2010	−43%
Saudi Arabia	2000	2015	−30%
Sweden	1996	2007	−50%
United Kingdom	1994–1998	2010	−40%
United States	1996	2008	−20%

[a] It should be noted that some of these targets also include reductions in serious injury and are supplemented by other targets, e.g. to reduce the numbers of casualties among children.

Sources: references *48, 79*.

of it into 30 km/h zones. A second phase of the programme will extend to 2010.

The Institute for Road Safety Research has estimated that an annual return on investment for the scheme of 9% will be forthcoming, which represents around twice the usual return of 4% from other large infrastructure projects.

Setting targets

Since the late 1980s, several countries have recognized that targets in road safety plans can be a useful tool for promoting proven casualty reduction measures higher up the list of political priorities, and for helping to attract appropriate resources for them. Many countries have set targets to reduce road casualties, and some of these are shown in Table 1.4.

International experience with numerical targets in road safety programmes, documented by

the Organisation for Economic Co-operation and Development (OECD) (*80*) and more recently by Elvik (*81*) and ETSC (*48*), indicates that setting quantitative targets can lead to better programmes, more effective use of resources and an improvement in road safety performance. A prerequisite for target setting is the availability of data on deaths and injuries, as well as information on traffic trends.

Elvik concluded that ambitious, long-term targets set by national governments appear to be the most effective in improving road safety performance (*81*).

Targets must be quantitative, time-dependent, easily intelligible and possible to evaluate. Among their main purposes are:

— to provide a rational means for identifying and carrying out interventions;
— to motivate those working in road safety;

— to raise the level of commitment to safety in the wider community;

— to encourage the ranking of safety measures (and their implementation) according to their value in reducing casualties;

— to encourage authorities with responsibilities for road safety to set their own targets;

— to allow assessments at different stages of a programme and to identify the scope for further activity.

Setting challenging but achievable road safety targets – something being done by an increasing number of countries – is a sign of responsible management. All the same, there is no guarantee that simply by setting targets, road safety performance will improve (81). In addition to a target, realistic safety programmes must be developed, properly implemented and well monitored. A survey undertaken of national road safety plans showed that planners need to consider (82):

— how to balance the objectives of safety, mobility and environmental concern;

— what barriers exist to implementing interventions, and how these could be overcome;

— how meaningful accountability for the achievement of goals could be obtained.

Policy-makers setting targets for higher safety levels need to concern themselves with a wide range of factors that influence safety (78, 83).

In New Zealand, the road traffic strategy sets four levels of target.

• The overall target is to reduce the socioeconomic costs of road crashes (including direct and indirect costs).

• This should be achieved by meeting the second level of targets, requiring specific reductions in the numbers of fatalities and serious injuries.

• A third level of targets consists of performance indicators (including those related to speed, drink driving and rates of seat-belt wearing) that are consistent with the targeted reductions in final outcomes.

• A fourth level of targets is concerned with institutional delivery outputs (such as the number of police patrol hours and the kilometres of

high-risk crash sites treated) that are required to achieve the third-level targets (25, 83, 84).

Partnerships in the public and private sectors

Significant progress has been made in establishing different types of partnerships within tiers of government and between the private and public sector. Some examples of effective partnerships are set out below.

The model of Victoria, Australia

The Australian state of Victoria has developed a strong partnership between traffic law enforcement and traffic injury compensation schemes, underpinned by the use of research to provide evidence for new policies and practices. In this scheme, the Transport Accidents Commission (TAC), set up in 1986, compensates victims of road crashes through a no-fault system (in which the insurer pays for any damages incurred in a crash, regardless of which party was considered at fault), funded by premiums that are levied as part of the annual vehicle registration charge.

The TAC determined that a substantial investment in road injury prevention would be more than offset by reduced payments in compensation. It invested heavily in the road agency's remedial programme for high-risk crash sites. It also helped the police purchase enforcement technology so as to raise levels of enforcement, and it embarked on an intense series of public education campaigns. The three separate ministries of the state government – those of transport, insurance and justice – jointly set policy and coordinated the programme.

A series of controlled enforcement and education programmes was undertaken, each subject to scientific evaluation. Victoria has a tradition of scientific evaluation of road safety interventions and enforcement practice, in particular, has in the past been shaped by research findings (85). An example is Victoria's approach to the enforcement of speed limits using speed cameras. In most other places, speed cameras are generally sited at crash "black spots", with signs and other overt signals maximizing the focus on the specific site. In Victoria, the objective, at least in urban areas, is to cover the whole road network. The strategy is thus covert and random – and, to the motorist, unpredictable. The link here between research and road safety policy-making is strong – making the intervention more effective. Since the potential benefits of the programme are scientifically researched and publicized, there is public support for the programme. This support may not otherwise have been forthcoming, as the seemingly draconian levels of enforcement might have led to public opposition.

The Victorian model has been adapted and implemented in South Africa's KwaZulu-Natal province – an example of a successful transfer of technology from a high-income country (86).

Safety partnerships in the United Kingdom

In 1998, the United Kingdom's Department for Transport, together with other government departments, created a policy of allowing local multisectoral partnerships, subject to strict financial criteria, to recover the costs of speed enforcement. The national project brought in representatives from a wide range of government and professional sectors.

In April 2000, pilot studies were launched in eight areas. The core membership of the partnerships included local authorities, the local law courts, the Highways Agency and the police. Some pilot areas also actively involved their local health sector organizations.

In those pilot studies where comparisons could be made, there was a 35% reduction in road crashes compared with the long-term trend during the first two years of the schemes, and a 56% reduction in fatal and serious pedestrian casualties (87).

The introduction of the cost recovery system has been a good example of "joined-up" government – seamless partnerships across a range of sectors – at both a national and local level. The process has enabled a more consistent and rigorous approach to enforcement, and it has freed up resources to focus on locally-targeted routes. In total, the system has released around £20 million of additional funds for local partnerships to spend on speed and traffic signal enforcement and on raising public awareness of the dangers of speeding. The benefits to society, in terms of casualties saved, have been estimated at around £112 million in the first two years of operation (87).

New car assessment programmes

People buying cars are becoming increasingly aware of the importance of safe car design and they frequently seek reliable information about the safety performance of individual car models. New Car Assessment Programmes (NCAPs) in which new car models are subjected to a range of crash tests and their performance rated with a "star" system have been developed around the world. Such programmes provide a resource for consumers, promote safety and also give credit to the efforts of car manufacturers that focus on safety. The first NCAP was set up in 1978 in the United States, followed by the Australian NCAP in 1992 and the European version (EuroNCAP) in 1996.

The EuroNCAP illustrates how a partnership between government, and motoring and consumer organizations can deliver an important source of impartial information about the performance of new cars in realistic crash tests. EuroNCAP's contributing organizations include the departments of transport of France, Germany, the Netherlands, Spain (Catalonia), Sweden and the United Kingdom. Also participating are the Allgemeiner Deutscher Automobil-Club (ADAC), the European Commission, the FIA Foundation, and – on behalf of European consumer organizations – the International Consumer Research and Testing (ICRT).

Types of whole vehicle tests (such as frontal impact, side impact and pedestrian-friendliness) and test procedures (including velocity, ground clearance height and percentage overlap tests) vary across the various NCAPs, making the comparison of systems based on crash tests more difficult.

Such information on the crash-worthiness of vehicles has helped consumers realize the value of safety and take the information into account when they purchase new vehicles. The car industry has consequently responded by making substantial improvements in car design over and above legislative requirements. However, there has been little response to date to the pedestrian protection tests undertaken in the Australian and European programmes. Research has shown that cars with three or four stars are approximately 30% safer, compared with two-star cars or cars without a Euro-NCAP score, in car-to-car collisions (*88*).

A promising similar development, led by the automobile clubs in Europe, ———— ———— ———— star rating system for specifi— ———— road builders are also enco— ———— safety of their roads beyond— ————

Conclusion

Road traffic injuries and d— ———— health issue worldwide. U— ———— is taken urgently, the probl— ———— This will particularly be th— ———— ing countries where rapid— ———— occur over the next two d— ———— of the burden of injury v— ———— by vulnerable road users – ———— motorcyclists.

There is hope, though, that the devastating loss of life and health entailed in such a worsening scenario can be avoided. Over the last forty years the science of traffic safety has developed to a point where the effective strategies for preventing or reducing crashes and injuries are well known.

A scientific, systems approach to the problem of road safety is essential, though it is not yet fully accepted in many places. The new model of understanding road safety can be summarized as follows:

- Crash injury is largely predictable and largely preventable. It is a problem amenable to rational analysis and remedy.
- Road safety policy must be based on a sound analysis and interpretation of data, rather than on anecdote.
- Road safety is a public health issue that intimately involves a range of sectors, including that of health. All have their responsibilities and all need to be fully engaged in injury prevention.
- Since human error in complex traffic systems cannot be eliminated entirely, environmental solutions (including the design of roads and

of vehicles) must help in making road traffic systems safer.
- The vulnerability of the human body should be a limiting design factor for traffic systems, i.e. for vehicle and road design, and for setting speed limits.
- Road crash injury is a social equity issue, with vulnerable road users bearing a dispro— ———— ———— —re of road injury and risk. The ———— al protection.
———— from high-income to ———— s must be appropriate ———— local needs, as deter—

———— eeds to feed in to the ———— ocal solutions.
———— dable challenge of reduc— ———— oss on the roads requires ———— oped:
———— ty for policy-making, ———— ventions, in both the pub— ———— tors;
— national strategic plans, incorporating targets where data allow;
— good data systems for identifying problems and evaluating responses;
— collaboration across a range of sectors, including the health sector;
— partnerships between public and private sectors;
— accountability, adequate resources and a strong political will.

References

1. Kopits E, Cropper M. *Traffic fatalities and economic growth*. Washington, DC, The World Bank, 2003 (Policy Research Working Paper No. 3035).

2. Murray CJL, Lopez AD, eds. *The global burden of disease: a comprehensive assessment of mortality and disability from diseases, injuries, and risk factors in 1990 and projected to 2020*. Boston, MA, Harvard School of Public Health, 1996.

3. *The world health report 2001. Mental health: new understanding, new hope*. Geneva, World Health Organization, 2001.

4. Peden M, McGee K, Sharma G. *The injury chart book: a graphical overview of the global burden of injuries.* Geneva, World Health Organization, 2002 (http://www.who.int/violence_injury_prevention/injury/chartbook/chartb/en/, accessed 30 October 2003).

5. Jacobs G, Aeron-Thomas A, Astrop A. *Estimating global road fatalities.* Crowthorne, Transport Research Laboratory, 2000 (TRL Report, No. 445).

6. Peden M, McGee K, Krug E, eds. *Injury: a leading cause of the global burden of disease, 2000.* Geneva, World Health Organization, 2002 (http://whqlibdoc.who.int/publications/2002/9241562323.pdf, accessed 30 October 2003).

7. Nantulya VM, Reich MR. The neglected epidemic: road traffic injuries in developing countries. *British Medical Journal,* 2002, 324: 1139–1141.

8. Nantulya VM et al. The global challenge of road traffic injuries: can we achieve equity in safety? *Injury Control and Safety Promotion,* 2003, 10:3–7.

9. *Transport safety performance in the EU: a statistical overview.* Brussels, European Transport Safety Council, 2003.

10. Murray CJL et al. *The Global Burden of Disease 2000 project: aims, methods and data sources* [revised]. Geneva, World Health Organization, 2001 (GPE Discussion Paper No. 36).

11. Gururaj G, Thomas AA, Reddi MN. Underreporting road traffic injuries in Bangalore: implications for road safety policies and programmes. In: *Proceedings of the 5th World Conference on Injury Prevention and Control.* New Delhi, Macmillan India, 2000:54 (Paper 1-3-I-04).

12. Varghese M, Mohan D. Transportation injuries in rural Haryana, North India. In: *Proceedings of the International Conference on Traffic Safety.* New Delhi, Macmillan India, 2003:326–329.

13. Mohan D. Traffic safety and health in Indian cities. *Journal of Transport and Infrastructure,* 2002, 9: 79–92.

14. Martinez R. Traffic safety as a health issue. In: von Holst H, Nygren A, Thord R, eds. *Traffic safety, communication and health.* Stockholm, Temaplan AB, 1996.

15. Evans L. *Traffic safety and the driver.* New York, NY, Van Nostrand Reinhold, 1991.

16. Mock CN et al. Incidence and outcome of injury in Ghana: a community-based survey. *Bulletin of the World Health Organization,* 1999, 77: 955–964.

17. London J et al. Using mortuary statistics in the development of an injury surveillance system in Ghana. *Bulletin of the World Health Organization,* 2002, 80:357–362.

18. Mock CN et al. Long-term injury-related disability in Ghana. *Disability and Rehabilitation,* 2003, 25:732–741.

19. Odero W, Garner P, Zwi A. Road traffic injuries in developing countries: a comprehensive review of epidemiological studies. *Tropical Medicine and International Health,* 1997, 2:445–460.

20. Barss P et al. *Injury prevention: an international perspective.* New York, NY, Oxford University Press, 1998.

21. *Transport accident costs and the value of safety.* Brussels, European Transport Safety Council, 1997.

22. Blincoe LJ et al. *The economic impact of motor vehicle crashes 2000.* Washington, DC, National Highway Traffic Safety Administration, 2002 (Report No. DOT HS-809-446).

23. Odero W, Khayesi M, Heda PM. Road traffic injuries in Kenya: magnitude, cause and status of intervention. *Injury Control and Safety Promotion,* 2003, 10:53–61.

24. Ad Hoc Committee on Health Research Relating to Future Intervention Options. *Investing in health research and development.* Geneva, World Health Organization, 1996 (TDR/Gen/96.2).

25. Koornstra M et al. *Sunflower: a comparative study of the development of road safety in Sweden, the United Kingdom and the Netherlands.* Leidschendam, Institute for Road Safety Research, 2002.

26. Roberts I, Mohan D, Abbasi K. War on the roads [Editorial]. *British Medical Journal,* 2002, 324:1107–1108.

27. Allsop R. *Road safety: Britain in Europe.* London, Parliamentary Advisory Council for Transport Safety, 2001 (http://www.pacts.org.uk/richardslecture.htm, accessed 30 October 2003).

28. Waters H, Hyder AA, Phillips T. Economic evaluation of interventions to reduce road traffic

injuries: with applications to low and middle-income countries. *Asia Pacific Journal of Public Health*, in press.

29. *Road traffic accidents: epidemiology, control and prevention.* Geneva, World Health Organization, 1962.

30. Loimer H, Guarnieri M. Accidents and acts of God: a history of terms. *American Journal of Public Health*, 1996, 86:101–107.

31. Nader R. *Unsafe at any speed*, 2nd ed. New York, NY, Grossman Publishers, 1972.

32. Haddon Jr W. The changing approach to the epidemiology, prevention, and amelioration of trauma: the transition to approaches etiologically rather than descriptively. *American Journal of Public Health*, 1968, 58:1431–1438.

33. Henderson M. Science and society. *Recovery*, 1996, 7:28–29.

34. Trinca GW et al. *Reducing traffic injury: the global challenge.* Melbourne, Royal Australasian College of Surgeons, 1988.

35. Mackay G. *Sharing responsibilities for road safety.* Brussels, European Transport Safety Council, 2001.

36. Sleet DA. Motor vehicle trauma and safety belt use in the context of public health priorities. *Journal of Trauma*, 1987, 27:695–702.

37. Henderson M, ed. *Public health and road safety: why can't we live with our roads?* [Conference proceedings of Australian Doctors' Fund and Royal Australasian College of Surgeons, "Keeping patients and doctors together", Sydney, 29–30 March 1990]. (http://www.adf.com.au/archive.php?doc_id=22, accessed 30 October 2003).

38. Waller P. Public health's contribution to motor vehicle injury prevention. *American Journal of Preventive Medicine*, 2001, 21(Suppl. 4):3–4.

39. Mackay GM. *Safer transport in Europe: tools for decision-making* [2nd European Transport Safety Lecture]. Brussels, European Transport Safety Council, 2000 (http://www.etsc.be/eve.htm, accessed 30 October 2003).

40. Nantulya VM, Reich MR. Equity dimensions of road traffic injuries in low- and middle-income countries. *Injury Control and Safety Promotion*, 2003, 10:13–20.

41. Laflamme L, Diderichsen F. Social differences in traffic injury risks in childhood and youth: a literature review and research agenda. *Injury Prevention*, 2000, 6:293–298.

42. Hippesley-Cox J et al. Cross sectional survey of socio-economic variations in severity and mechanism of childhood injuries in Trent 1992–97. *British Medical Journal*, 2002, 324:1132–1134.

43. Hasselberg M, Laflamme L, Ringback Wetoft G. Socio-economic differences in road traffic during childhood and youth: a closer look at different kinds of road user. *Journal of Epidemiology and Community Health*, 2001, 55:858–862.

44. Mock CN, nii-Amon-Kotei D, Maier RV. Low utilization of formal medical services by injured persons in a developing nation: health service data underestimate the importance of trauma. *Journal of Trauma*, 1997, 42:504–513.

45. Hijar M, Vazquez-Vela E, Arreola-Risa C. Pedestrian traffic injuries in Mexico: a country update. *Injury Control and Safety Promotion*, 2003, 10:37–43.

46. Ghaffar A et al. The burden of road traffic injuries in developing countries: the 1st National Injury Survey of Pakistan. *Public Health*, in press.

47. *International Road Traffic and Accident Database* [web site]. Paris, Organisation for Economic Co-operation and Development, 2003 (http://www.bast.de/IRTAD, accessed 30 October 2003).

48. *Risk assessment and target setting in EU transport programmes.* Brussels, European Transport Safety Council, 2003.

49. Mohan D. Road safety in less-motorised environment: future concerns. *International Journal of Epidemiology*, 2002, 31:527–532.

50. Mohan D, Tiwari G. Traffic safety in low income countries: issues and concerns regarding technology transfer from high-income countries. In: *Reflections of the transfer of traffic safety knowledge to motorising nations.* Melbourne, Global Traffic Safety Trust, 1998:27–56.

51. Nantulya VM, Muli-Musiime F. Uncovering the social determinants of road traffic accidents in Kenya. In: Evans T et al, eds. *Challenging inequities: from ethics to action.* Oxford, Oxford University Press, 2001:211–225.

52. Rumar K. *Transport safety visions, targets and strategies: beyond 2000*. [1st European Transport Safety Lecture]. Brussels, European Transport Safety Council, 1999 (http://www.etsc.be/eve.htm, accessed 30 October 2003).

53. Duperrex O, Bunn F, Roberts I. Safety education of pedestrians for injury prevention: a systematic review of randomised controlled trials. *British Medical Journal*, 2002, 324:1129–1133.

54. Reason J. *Human error*. Cambridge, Cambridge University Press, 1990.

55. Tingvall C. The Zero Vision. In: van Holst H, Nygren A, Thord R, eds. *Transportation, traffic safety and health: the new mobility. Proceedings of the 1st International Conference Gothenburg, Sweden, 1995*. Berlin, Springer-Verlag, 1995:35–57.

56. O'Neill B, Mohan D. Reducing motor vehicle crash deaths and injuries in newly motorising countries. *British Medical Journal*, 2002, 324: 1142–1145.

57. *En route to a society with safe road traffic*. Stockholm, Swedish Ministry of Transport and Communication, 1997 (Memorandum DS).

58. Wegman F, Elsenaar P. *Sustainable solutions to improve road safety in the Netherlands*. Leidschendam, Institute for Road Safety Research, 1997 (SWOV Report D-097-8).

59. Belin MA et al. The vision zero and its consequences. In: *Proceedings of the 4th International Conference on Safety and the Environment in the 21st Century, Tel Aviv, Israel, 23–27 November 1997*. Haifa, Transportation Research Institute, 1997:1–14.

60. Mackay GM. Reducing car crash injuries, folklore, science and promise. *American Association for Automotive Medicine Quarterly Journal*, 1983, 5: 27–32.

61. Tingvall C, Haworth N. *Vision Zero: an ethical approach to safety and mobility*. [Paper presented to the 6th Institute of Transport Engineers International Conference on Road Safety and Traffic Enforcement: Beyond 2000, Melbourne, 6–7 September 1999] (http://www.general.monash.edu.au/MUARC/viszero.htm, accessed 30 October 2003).

62. Mohan D, Tiwari G. Road safety in less motorised countries: relevance of international vehi-

cle and highway safety standards. In: *Proceedings of the International Conference on Vehicle Safety 2000*. London, Institution of Mechanical Engineers, 2000:155–166.

63. Tiwari G. Traffic flow and safety: need for new models in heterogeneous traffic: In: Mohan D, Tiwari G, eds. *Injury prevention and control*. London, Taylor & Francis, 2000:71–88.

64. Whitelegg J, Haq G. The global transport problem: same issues but a different place. In: Whitelegg J, Haq G, eds. *The Earthscan reader on world transport, policy and practice*. London, Earthscan Publications, 2003:1–28.

65. *Reflections on the transfer of traffic safety knowledge to motorising nations*. Melbourne, Global Traffic Safety Trust, 1998.

66. Johnston I. Traffic safety in a developmental context. In: *Reflections on the transfer of traffic safety knowledge to motorising nations*. Melbourne, Global Traffic Safety Trust, 1998:7–13.

67. Forjuoh SN. Traffic-related injury prevention interventions for low-income countries. *Injury Control and Safety Promotion*, 2003, 10:109–118.

68. Rothe JP, ed. *Driving lessons: exploring systems that make traffic safer*. Edmonton, University of Alberta Press, 2002.

69. Centers for Disease Control and Prevention. Motor vehicle safety: a 20th century public health achievement. *Morbidity and Mortality Weekly Report*, 1999, 48:369–374.

70. Lonero L et al. *Road safety as a social construct*. Ottawa, Northport Associates, 2002 (Transport Canada Report No. 8080-00-1112).

71. Wesemann P. *Economic evaluation of road safety measures*. Leidschendam, Institute for Road Safety Research, 2000 (SWOV Report D-2000-16E).

72. Aeron-Thomas A et al. *A review of road safety management and practice. Final report*. Crowthorne, Transport Research Laboratory and Babtie Ross Silcock, 2002 (TRL Report PR/INT216/2002).

73. Heiman L. *Vehicle occupant protection in Australia*. Canberra, Federal Office of Road Safety, 1988.

74. Hyder AA. Health research investments: a challenge for national public health associations. *Journal of the Pakistan Medical Association*, 2002, 52: 276–277.

75. Hyder AA, Akhter T, Qayyum A. Capacity development for health research in Pakistan: the effect of doctoral training. *Health Policy and Planning*, 2003, 18:338–343.

76. Russell-Bolen J, Sleet DA, Johnson V, eds. *Prevention of motor vehicle-related injuries: a compendium of articles from the Morbidity and Mortality Weekly Report, 1985–1996*. Atlanta, GA, United States Department of Health and Human Services, Centers for Disease Control and Prevention, 1997.

77. Breen J. Promoting research-based road safety policies in Europe: the role of the non-governmental sector. In: *Proceedings of the 2nd European Road Research Conference*. Brussels, European Commission, 1999 (http://europea.eu.int/comm/transport/road/research/2nd_errc/contents/15%20SAFETY%20RESEARCH/safety%20research%20pol.doc, accessed 30 October 2003).

78. *Transport safety performance indicators*. Brussels, European Transport Safety Council, 2001.

79. Elvik R, Vaa T. *Handbook of road safety measures*. Amsterdam, Elsevier, in press.

80. *Targeted road safety programmes*. Paris, Organisation for Economic Co-operation and Development, 1994.

81. Elvik R. *Quantified road safety targets: an assessment of evaluation methodology*. Oslo, Institute of Transport Economics, 2001 (Report No. 539).

82. Johnston I. Action to reduce road casualties. *World Health Forum*, 1992, 13:154–162.

83. Bliss A. *Road safety in the developing world*. [Paper presented at the World Bank Transport Forum, Session 2–2: health sector linkages with transport.] Washington, DC, The World Bank, 2003 (http://www.worldbank.org/transport/forum2003/presentations/bliss.ppt, accessed 30 October 2003).

84. *Road safety strategy 2010: a consultation document*. Wellington, Land Transport Safety Authority, 2000.

85. Delaney A. Diamantopolou K, Cameron M. *MUARC's speed enforcement research: principles learnt and implications for practice*. Melbourne, Monash University Accident Research Centre, 2003 (Report No. 200).

86. Spencer TJ. The Victoria model in Kwazulu-Natal. *Joint Economic Commission for Africa/Organisation for Economic Co-operation and Development. Third African road safety congress. Compendium of papers, volume 1. 14–17 April 1997, Pretoria, South Africa*. Addis Ababa, Economic Commission for Africa, 1997:153–169.

87. Gains A et al. *A cost recovery system for speed and red light cameras – two-year pilot evaluation*. London, Department for Transport, 2003.

88. Lie A, Tingvall C. How do Euro NCAP results correlate with real-life injury risks? A paired comparison study of car-to-car crashes. *Traffic Injury Prevention*, 2002, 3:288–291.

CHAPTER 2

The global impact

Introduction

The previous chapter showed that road traffic injuries are a major global public health and development problem that will worsen in the years ahead if no significant steps are taken to alleviate it. This chapter examines in greater depth the extent of the problem of road traffic injuries. The current global estimates and trends over time are first discussed, with projections and predictions. The sections that follow examine the effects of motorization, the profiles of those affected by road traffic injuries, and the socioeconomic and health impacts of road traffic collisions. Finally, there is a discussion of important issues related to data and the evidence for road traffic injury prevention.

Sources of data

The analysis in this chapter is based on evidence on road traffic injuries derived from four main sources:

- The WHO mortality database and the WHO Global Burden of Disease (GBD), 2002, Version 1 database (see Statistical Annex).
- Recent studies by the World Bank (1) and the United Kingdom's Transport Research Laboratory (now TRL Ltd) (2).
- Databases and web sites of various international and national organizations that compile road transport statistics, including:
  - International Road Traffic and Accident Database (IRTAD);
  - United Nations Economic Commission for Europe (UNECE);
  - Transport Safety Bureau, Australia.
  - Department of Transport, South Africa;
  - Department for Transport, United Kingdom;
  - Fatal Analysis Reporting System, United States;
  - National Highway Traffic Safety Administration (NHTSA), United States;
- A review of available studies on various topics related to road traffic injuries, including road safety issues, in order to secure country and regional level data and evidence. The literature was obtained from libraries, online journals and individuals.

Magnitude of the problem

Mortality is an essential indicator of the scale of any health problem, including injury. It is important, though, that non-fatal outcomes – or injury morbidity – should be measured and included, so as to reflect fully the burden of disease due to road traffic collisions. For each road traffic injury death, there are dozens of survivors who are left with short-term or permanent disabilities that may result in continuing restrictions on their physical functioning, psychosocial consequences or a reduced quality of life. The assessment in this chapter of the magnitude of road traffic injuries, therefore, considers not only on mortality but also injuries and disability.

Global estimates

The road traffic injury problem began before the introduction of the car. However, it was with the car – and subsequently buses, trucks and other vehicles – that the problem escalated rapidly. By various accounts, the first injury crash was supposedly suffered by a cyclist in New York City on 30 May 1896, followed a few months later by the first fatality, a pedestrian in London (3). Despite the early concerns expressed over serious injury and loss of life, road traffic crashes have continued to this day to exact their toll. Though the exact number will never be known, the number of fatalities was conservatively estimated to have reached a cumulative total of 25 million by 1997 (4).

WHO data show that in 2002 nearly 1.2 million people worldwide died as a result of road traffic injuries (see Statistical Annex, Table A.2). This represents an average of 3242 persons dying each day around the world from road traffic injuries. In addition to these deaths, between 20 million and 50 million people globally are estimated to be injured or disabled each year (2, 5, 6).

In the same year, the overall global road traffic injury mortality rate was 19.0 per 100 000 population (see Table 2.1). Low-income and middle-income countries had a rate slightly greater than the global average, while that for high-income countries was considerably lower. The vast majority – 90% – of road traffic deaths were in low-income and middle-income countries. Only 10% of road traffic deaths occurred in high-income countries.

TABLE 2.1

Estimated global road traffic injury-related deaths

	Number	Rate per 100 000 population	Proportion of total (%)
Low-income and middle-income countries	1 065 988	20.2	90
High-income countries	117 504	12.6	10
Total	1 183 492	19.0	100

Source: WHO Global Burden of Disease project, 2002, Version 1 (see Statistical Annex).

According to WHO data for 2002, road traffic injuries accounted for 2.1% of all global deaths (see Statistical Annex, Table A.2) and ranked as the 11th leading cause of death (see Statistical Annex, Table A.3). Furthermore, these road traffic deaths accounted for 23% of all injury deaths worldwide (see Figure 2.1).

FIGURE 2.1

Distribution of global injury mortality by cause

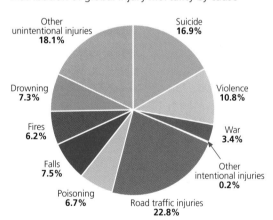

Source: WHO Global Burden of Disease project, 2002, Version 1 (see Statistical Annex).

In 2002, road traffic injuries were the ninth leading cause of disability-adjusted life years lost (see Statistical Annex, Table A.3), accounting for over 38 million disability-adjusted life years (DALYs) lost, or 2.6% of the global burden of disease. Low-income and middle-income countries account for 91.8% of the DALYs lost to road traffic injuries worldwide.

These observations illustrate the fact that low-income and middle-income countries carry most of the burden of the world's road traffic injuries.

Regional distribution

There is considerable regional variation, both in the absolute number of road traffic injury deaths and mortality rates (see Statistical Annex, Table A.2). The WHO Western Pacific Region recorded the highest absolute number of deaths in 2002, with just over 300 000, followed by the WHO South-East Asia Region with just under 300 000. These two regions together account for more than half of all road traffic deaths in the world.

As regards death rates, the WHO African Region had the highest mortality rate in 2002, at 28.3 per 100 000 population, followed closely by the low-income and middle-income countries of the WHO Eastern Mediterranean Region, at 26.4 per 100 000 population (see Figure 2.2 and Table 2.2).

TABLE 2.2

Road traffic injury mortality rates (per 100 000 population) in WHO regions, 2002

WHO region	Low-income and middle-income countries	High-income countries
African Region	28.3	—
Region of the Americas	16.2	14.8
South-East Asia Region	18.6	—
European Region	17.4	11.0
Eastern Mediterranean Region	26.4	19.0
Western Pacific Region	18.5	12.0

Source: WHO Global Burden of Disease project, 2002, Version 1 (see Statistical Annex).

The high-income countries in Europe have the lowest road traffic fatality rate (11.0 per 100 000 population) followed by those of the WHO Western Pacific Region (12.0 per 100 000 population). In general, the regional averages for low-income and middle-income are much higher than corresponding rates for high-income countries.

Significant variations also arise between countries; some features specific to individual countries are discussed below.

FIGURE 2.2

Road traffic injury mortality rates (per 100 000 population) in WHO regions, 2002

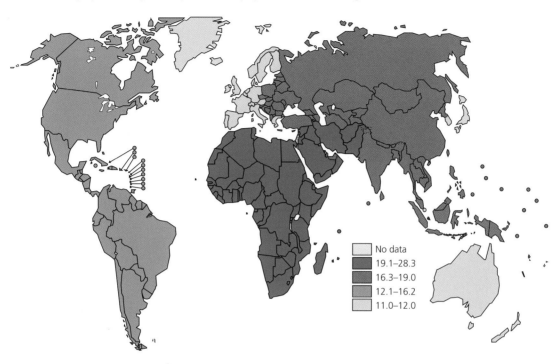

No data
19.1–28.3
16.3–19.0
12.1–16.2
11.0–12.0

Source: WHO Global Burden of Disease project, 2002, Version 1 (see Statistical Annex).

Country estimates

Only 75 countries report vital registration data, including road traffic injury data, to WHO that are sufficient for analysis here (see Statistical Annex, Table A.4). The regional estimates, presented in the section above, are based on these data, as well as on incomplete data from a further 35 countries and various epidemiological sources. These estimates indicate that African countries have some of the highest road traffic injury mortality rates. However, when examining data from the individual 75 countries that report sufficient data to WHO, a different picture emerges. The highest country rates are found in some Latin American countries (41.7 per 100 000 population in El Salvador, 41.0 per 100 000 in the Dominican Republic and 25.6 per 100 000 in Brazil), as well as some countries in Europe (22.7 per 100 000 in Latvia, 19.4 per 100 000 in the Russian Federation and 19.3 per 100 000 in Lithuania), and Asia (21.9 per 100 000 in the Republic of Korea, 21.0 per 100 000 in Thailand and 19.0 per 100 000 in China).

Many Member countries of the Organisation for Economic Co-operation and Development (OECD) report road traffic fatality rates of less than 10 per 100 000 population (see Table 2.3). The Netherlands, Sweden and Great Britain have the lowest rates per 100 000 population.

TABLE 2.3

Road traffic fatality rates in selected countries or areas, 2000

Country or area	Per 100 000 inhabitants
Australia	9.5
European Union[a]	11.0
Great Britain	5.9
Japan	8.2
Netherlands	6.8
Sweden	6.7
United States of America	15.2

[a] Austria, Belgium, Denmark, Finland, France, Germany, Greece, Ireland, Italy, Luxembourg, Netherlands, Portugal, Spain, Sweden and the United Kingdom.

Source: reproduced from reference 7, with minor editorial amendments, with the permission of the publisher.

Trends in road traffic injuries
Global and regional trends

According to WHO data, road traffic deaths have risen from approximately 999 000 in 1990 (*8*) to just over 1.1 million in 2002 (see Statistical Annex, Table A.2) – an increase of around 10%. Low-income and middle-income countries account for the majority of this increase.

Although the number of road traffic injuries has continued to rise in the world as a whole, time series analysis reveals that road traffic fatalities and mortality rates show clear differences in the pattern of growth between high-income countries, on the one hand, and low-income and middle-income countries on the other (*2, 9–11*). In general, since the 1960s and 1970s, there has been a decrease in the numbers and rates of fatalities in high-income countries such as Australia, Canada, Germany, the Netherlands, Sweden, the United Kingdom and the United States of America. At the same time, there has been a pronounced rise in numbers and rates in many low-income and middle-income countries.

The percentage change in road traffic fatalities in different regions of the world for the period 1987–1995 is shown in Figure 2.3. The trends are based on a limited number of countries for which data were available throughout the period and they are therefore influenced by the largest countries in the regional samples. Such regional trends could mask national trends and the data should not be extrapolated to the national level. The regional classifications employed are similar to, but not exactly the same as those defined by WHO. It is clear from the figure that there has been an overall downward trend in road traffic deaths in high-income countries, whereas many of the low-income and middle-income countries have shown an increase since the late 1980s. There are, however, some marked regional differences; Central and Eastern Europe witnessed a rapid increase in road traffic deaths during the late 1980s, the rate of increase of which has since declined. The onset of rapid increases in road traffic fatalities occurred later in Latin America and the Caribbean, from 1992 onwards. In contrast, numbers of road traffic deaths have risen steadily

since the late 1980s in the Middle East and North Africa and in Asia, particularly in the former.

The reductions in road traffic fatalities in high-income countries are attributed largely to the implementation of a wide range of road safety measures, including seat-belt use, vehicle crash protection, traffic-calming interventions and traffic law enforcement (*2, 12*). However, the reduction in the reported statistics for road traffic injury does not necessarily mean an improvement in road safety for everyone. According to the International Road Traffic and Accident Database (IRTAD), pedestrian and bicyclist fatalities have decreased more rapidly than have fatalities among vehicle occupants. In fact, between 1970 and 1999, the proportion of pedestrian and bicyclist fatalities fell from 37% to 25% of all traffic fatalities, when averaged across 28 countries that report their data to IRTAD (*13*). These reductions could, however, be due, at least in part, to a decrease in exposure rather than an improvement in safety (*14*).

FIGURE 2.3

Global and regional road fatality trends, 1987–1995[a]

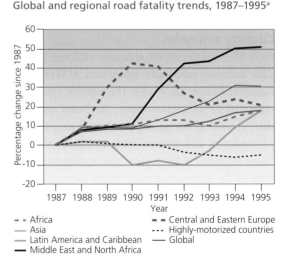

- - Africa
— Asia
— Latin America and Caribbean
— Middle East and North Africa
- - Central and Eastern Europe
--- Highly-motorized countries
— Global

[a] Data are displayed according to the regional classifications of TRL Ltd, United Kingdom.

Source: reproduced from reference *2* with the permission of the author.

Trends in selected countries

As already mentioned, the regional trends do not necessarily reflect those of individual countries.

Table 2.4 and Figures 2.4 and 2.5 show how road traffic mortality rates have changed with time in some countries. It can be seen from Figures 2.4 and 2.5 that some individual countries' trends in mortality rates do indeed reflect the general trend in the number of road traffic deaths. Thus in Australia, the mortality rate increased – with some annual fluctuations – to peak at about 30 deaths per 100 000 population in 1970, after which there was a steady decline. Trends in the United Kingdom and the United States followed a similar pattern. The rates in Brazil, on the other hand, appear to have reached a peak in 1981 and may now be declining very slowly. In contrast, India, with relatively high rates of population growth, increasing mobility and growing numbers of vehicles, is still

FIGURE 2.4

Road traffic fatality trends in three high-income countries (Australia, United Kingdom, United States of America)

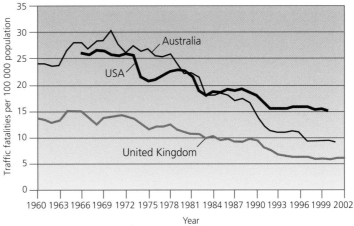

Sources: Transport Safety Bureau, Australia; Department of Transport; United Kingdom; Fatality Analysis Reporting System, United States of America.

TABLE 2.4

Changes in road traffic fatality rates
(deaths per 10 000 population), 1975–1998

Country or area	Change (%)
Canada	–63.4
China	
Hong Kong SAR	–61.7
Province of Taiwan	–32.0
Sweden	–58.3
Israel	–49.7
France	–42.6
New Zealand	–33.2
United States of America	–27.2
Japan	–24.5
Malaysia	44.3
India	79.3[a]
Sri Lanka	84.5
Lesotho	192.8
Colombia	237.1
China	243.0
Botswana	383.8[b]

SAR: Special Administrative Region.

[a] Refers to the period 1980–1998.

[b] Refers to the period 1976–1998.

Source: reproduced from reference 1, with minor editorial amendments, with the permission of the authors.

showing a rising trend in mortality rates.

There are many factors contributing to these trends and the differences between countries and regions. At the macro level, these trends have been successfully modelled and used for predicting future developments.

Projections and predictions

While a decrease in deaths has been recorded in high-income countries, current and projected trends in low-income and middle-income countries foreshadow a large escalation in global road traffic mortality over the next 20 years and possibly beyond. Currently, there are two main models for predicting future trends in road traffic fatalities. These two models are:

— the WHO Global Burden of Disease (GBD) project (8), using health data;

— the World Bank's Traffic Fatalities and Economic Growth (TFEC) project (1), using transport, population and economic data.

Both predict a substantial increase in road traffic deaths if present policies and actions in road safety continue and no additional road safety countermeasures are put into place. The GBD model predicts the following scenario for 2020 compared with 1990 (8):

FIGURE 2.5

Road traffic fatality trends in three low-income and middle-income countries

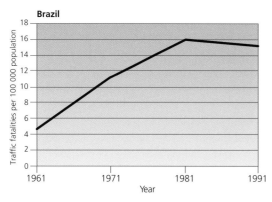

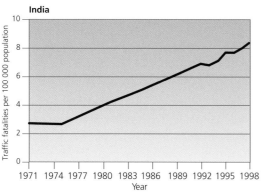

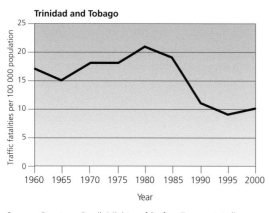

Sources: Denatran, Brazil; Ministry of Surface Transport, India; Police statistics, Highway Patrol Unit, Trinidad and Tobago Police Service.

- Road traffic injuries will rise in rank to sixth place as a major cause of death worldwide.
- Road traffic injuries will rise to become the third leading cause of DALYs lost.

- Road traffic injuries will become the second leading cause of DALYs lost for low-income and middle-income countries.
- Road traffic deaths will increase worldwide, from 0.99 million to 2.34 million (representing 3.4% of all deaths).
- Road traffic deaths will increase on average by over 80% in low-income and middle-income countries and decline by almost 30% in high-income countries.
- DALYs lost will increase worldwide from 34.3 million to 71.2 million (representing 5.1% of the global burden of disease).

FIGURE 2.6

Road traffic fatalities, adjusted for underreporting, 1990–2020

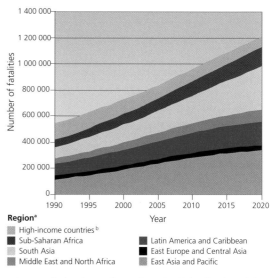

Region[a]

- High-income countries [b]
- Sub-Saharan Africa
- South Asia
- Middle East and North Africa
- Latin America and Caribbean
- East Europe and Central Asia
- East Asia and Pacific

[a] Data are displayed according to the regional classifications of the World Bank.
[b] 28 countries with a Human Development Index of 0.8 or more.
Source: reproduced from reference 1, with the permission of the authors.

According to the TFEC model predictions (Table 2.5 and Figure 2.6), between 2000 and 2020, South Asia will record the largest growth in road traffic deaths, with a dramatic increase of 144%. If the low-income and middle-income countries follow the general trend of the high-income countries, their fatality rates will begin to decline in the future, but not before costing many lives. The

TABLE 2.5

Predicted road traffic fatalities by region (in thousands), adjusted for underreporting, 1990–2020

Region[a]	Number of countries	1990	2000	2010	2020	Change (%) 2000–2020	Fatality rate (deaths/ 100 000 persons)	
							2000	2020
East Asia and Pacific	15	112	188	278	337	79	10.9	16.8
East Europe and Central Asia	9	30	32	36	38	19	19.0	21.2
Latin America and Caribbean	31	90	122	154	180	48	26.1	31.0
Middle East and North Africa	13	41	56	73	94	68	19.2	22.3
South Asia	7	87	135	212	330	144	10.2	18.9
Sub-Saharan Africa	46	59	80	109	144	80	12.3	14.9
Sub-total	121	419	613	862	1 124	83	13.3	19.0
High-income countries	35	123	110	95	80	−27	11.8	7.8
Total	156	542	723	957	1 204	67	13.0	17.4

[a] Data are displayed according to the regional classifications of the World Bank.

Source: reproduced from reference 1, with minor amendments, with the permission of the authors.

model anticipates that India's rate will not decline until 2042. Other low-income and middle-income country rates may begin to decline earlier, but their fatality rates will still be higher than those experienced by high-income countries.

The predicted percentage decrease in deaths from 2000 to 2020 for high-income countries of 27% and the global increase of 67% in the TFEC model are similar to those of the GBD model. However, the models differ on the total number of deaths each predicts for 2020. The TFEC model suggests that there will be 1.2 million deaths, as against 2.4 million for the GBD model. To some extent, this difference is explained by a much higher starting estimate for 1990 in the GBD model, which is based on data from health facilities.

The predictions need to be interpreted in context. The international data presented in this report show that at each income level, there are significant differences among countries in the number of vehicles per capita and in fatalities per capita. This implies that it is possible for people to live with fewer vehicles per capita and fewer fatalities per capita than the average rates seen at present. Projected trends are based on the averages of past trends. While existing scientific knowledge has not always been easily accessible for most countries, efforts are now being made to collate and disseminate this information so that it can be fed into predictive models. It is feasible, therefore, that low-

income and middle-income countries will not follow the trends of the past and even that they could improve upon them. As a result, the projections of the World Bank and WHO may prove too high and low-income and middle-income countries may see much lower death rates in the future.

Both models have made a large number of assumptions about the future and are based on scarce and imperfect data. Moreover, models cannot be expected to predict future reality precisely, as unforeseen factors will almost inevitably emerge. Nevertheless, the underlying message from the projections is clear: should current trends continue and no intensified and new interventions be implemented, then many more deaths and injuries will be experienced from road traffic crashes in the future. Helping low-income and middle-income countries tackle the problem of road traffic injuries must be a priority, as these are the countries where the greatest increases will occur in the next 20 years.

Motorization, development and road traffic injury

The earlier discussion on estimates and trends has shown that the road traffic injury problem is a complex one and represents the unfolding of many changes and events, both economic and social. The intricate relationship between road traffic injuries, motor vehicle numbers and a country's stage of development has been explored in a number of studies.

This section describes factors affecting trends in road traffic mortality rates, and, in particular, empirical findings on the links between road traffic fatalities, the growth in the number of motor vehicles and development.

The growth in the number of motor vehicles in various parts of the world is central, not only to road safety, but also to other issues such as pollution, the quality of life in urban and rural areas, the depletion of natural resources, and social justice (15–20).

As regards the number of fatalities, many high-income countries in the first half of the 20th century experienced a rapid growth in deaths from road crashes, alongside economic growth and an increase in the number of vehicles. During the second half of the century, though, many of these countries saw reductions in fatality rates, despite a continued rise in the number of motor vehicles and in mobility. It does not follow, therefore, that a growth in mobility and motorization will necessarily lead to higher rates of fatalities.

The first significant attempt to model the relationship between fatality rates and motorization was carried out by Smeed (21), who used data from 1938 for 20 industrialized countries. Smeed came to the conclusion that fatalities per motor vehicle decreased with an increasing number of vehicles per head of population. A similar relationship was later established for 32 developing countries, based on 1968 data (22). This research led to a basic belief that the road traffic injury death rate per registered vehicle is expected to decrease as the number of vehicles per head of population increases. However, this model was derived from a cross-section of countries and not from a time series of data for one or more countries. It is therefore dangerous to apply this model to changes over time in a single country. Furthermore, the use of the variable "fatalities per vehicle" has been criticized as an indicator for road traffic safety. It tends to ignore, for example, non-motorized forms of transport (23). Nor does it take into account other relevant road and environmental conditions, or the behaviour of drivers and other road users (24). The use of appropriate indicators for road safety is discussed in more detail later in this chapter.

Researchers have also investigated the relationship between road traffic injuries and other socioeconomic indicators (1, 25–29). For instance, it is known that the mortality rate, especially that of infant mortality, tends to improve as the gross national product (GNP) per capita increases. As a nation develops economically, it is to be expected that part of the wealth generated will be devoted to efforts to reduce mortality, including road traffic mortality (27). In this context, mortality related to motor vehicles and road traffic can be seen as a "disease of development".

A study of motor vehicle-related mortality in 46 countries (27) established a direct but weak correlation between economic development – as measured by GNP per capita – and deaths per vehicle. This relationship was found to be strongest among countries with low GNP per capita, yet it was precisely among these countries that the effects of factors other than GNP per capita on fatalities per vehicle were most important. Based on 1990 data, another study established a positive relationship between GNP per capita and road traffic mortality rates for 83 countries (29). In absolute terms, the middle-income countries had the highest mortality rates. When adjustments were made for the number of motor vehicles, the poorest countries showed the highest road traffic mortality rates.

A recent World Bank report (1) examined data from 1963 to 1999 for 88 countries. Unlike Smeed's research, the authors were able to develop models based on time series data for each country. One of their main findings was a sharp increase in fatalities per head of population as gross domestic product (GDP) per capita increased – but only at low levels of GDP per capita, up to a peak of between $6100 and $8600 (at 1985 international dollar values), depending on the exact model. After that peak was reached, fatalities per head of population began to decline. Their results also showed that fatalities per vehicle declined sharply with income per capita GDP in excess of $1180 (1985 international dollar values). The empirical results presented show the important contribution of economic development to mobility, which leads to increased motorization and increased exposure to risk.

Profile of people affected by road traffic injuries

Types of road user

Although all types of road user are at risk of being injured or killed in a road traffic crash, there are notable differences in fatality rates between different road user groups. In particular, the "vulnerable" road users such as pedestrians and two-wheeler users are at greater risk than vehicle occupants and usually bear the greatest burden of injury. This is especially true in low-income and middle-income countries, because of the greater variety and intensity of traffic mix and the lack of separation from other road users. Of particular concern is the mix between the slow-moving and vulnerable non-motorized road users, as well as motorcycles, and fast-moving, motorized vehicles.

Several studies have revealed marked differences in fatality rates between various groups of road users, as well as between road users in high-income countries and those in low-income and middle-income countries. A review of 38 studies found that pedestrian fatalities were highest in 75% of the studies, accounting for between 41% and 75% of all fatalities (30). Passengers were the second largest group of road users killed, accounting for between 38% and 51% of fatalities. In Kenya, between 1971 and 1990, pedestrians represented 42% of all crash fatalities; pedestrians and passengers combined accounted for approximately 80% of all fatalities in that country each year (31). In the city of Nairobi, between 1977 and 1994, 64% of road users killed in traffic crashes were pedestrians (32).

Recent studies have shown that pedestrians and motorcyclists have the highest rates of injury in Asia (33–35). Injured pedestrians and passengers in mass transportation are the main issue in Africa (31, 36, 37). In Latin America and the Caribbean, injuries to pedestrians are the greatest problem (38–40).

By contrast, in most OECD countries, such as France, Germany and Sweden, car occupants represent more than 60% of all fatalities, a reflection of the greater number of motor vehicles in use. While there are fewer motorcyclist, cyclist and pedestrian casualties, these groups of road users bear higher fatality rates (41).

In several low-income and middle-income countries, passengers in buses and other informal public transport systems also constitute a significant group at high risk of road traffic casualties (30) (see Box 2.1).

BOX 2.1

Informal types of transport

Public transport systems – such as buses, trains, underground trains and trams – are not well developed in many low-income and middle-income countries. Instead, informal modes of transport, used largely by poorer people, have evolved to fill the gap, consisting of privately-owned buses, converted pick-up trucks and minibuses. Examples include the *matatu* in Kenya, the light buses of Hong Kong and the minibuses of Singapore, Manila's *jeepneys*, the *colt* of Jakarta, the *dolmus* minibuses of Istanbul, the *dala dala* of Tanzania, the *tro-tro* of Ghana, the Haitian *tap-tap*, the *molue* (locally known as "moving morgues") and *danfo* ("flying coffins") in Nigeria, and the taxis of South Africa and Uganda (10).

The low fares charged by these forms of transport are affordable to poor people. The vehicles are also convenient, as they will stop anywhere to pick up or drop off passengers, and they do not adhere to any fixed time schedules. Against these advantages for poorer people in terms of mobility, there is a marked lack of safety. The vehicles are generally overloaded with passengers and goods. The drivers speed, are aggressive in their road behaviour and lack respect for other road users. The long hours that drivers are forced to work result in fatigue, sleep deprivation and reckless driving (42).

BOX 2.1 (continued)

These forms of transport thus present a real dilemma for road transport planners. On the one hand, the people who use them lack alternative safe and affordable public transport. These types of transport provide employment for poor people, and it is difficult to prohibit them. On the other hand, they are inherently dangerous. The drivers, subject to all-powerful vehicle owners, are not protected by labour laws. The owners frequently have their own private arrangements with the traffic enforcement authorities. All these factors increase the risk of vehicle crashes and injuries, and complicate possibilities for intervention.

All the same, a strategy must be found to regulate this industry and make it into a safe and organized form of public transport. Such a strategy must address the safety of road users, the labour rights of drivers and the economic interests of the vehicle owners (10, 42, 43). One possibility is that vehicle owners could be encouraged to pool their resources through some form of joint venture and be given access to additional capital and management capacity, so that a safe and effectively-regulated public transport system could be developed.

As Figure 2.7 shows, numerically, there are clear regional and national differences in the distribution of road user mortality. Vulnerable road users – pedestrians and cyclists – tend to account for a much greater proportion of road traffic deaths in low-income and middle-income countries, than in high-income countries. This is further illustrated in Table 2.6, which shows that pedestrians, cyclists and motorized two-wheeler riders sustain the vast majority of fatalities and injuries on both urban and rural roads.

The type of traffic, the mix of different types of road user, and the type of crashes in low-income and middle-income countries differ significantly from those in high-income countries. Their traffic patterns have generally not been experienced by high-income countries in the past and so technologies and policies cannot be automatically transferred from high-income to low-income countries without adaptation. A good example of this provided by that of Viet Nam, where rapid motorization has occurred as a result of the proliferation of small and inexpensive motorcycles. These motorcycles, whose number is likely

FIGURE 2.7

Road users killed in various modes of transport as a proportion of all road traffic deaths

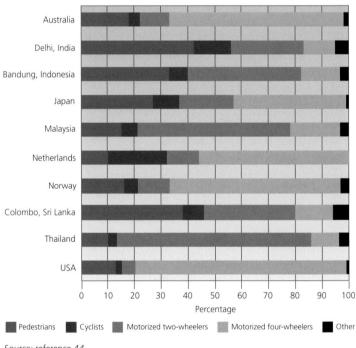

Source: reference 44.

to remain high, have recently been joined by a large influx of passenger motor vehicles, creating increased crash risks because of the mix of different types of road user.

In many low-income and middle-income countries, where bicycles and motorcycles are often the only affordable means of transport, two-wheeled

TABLE 2.6

Proportion of road users killed at different locations in India

Location	Type of road user (%)								
	Lorry	Bus	Car	TSR	MTW	HAPV	Bicycle	Pedestrian	Total
Mumbai	2	1	2	4	7	0	6	78	100
New Delhi	2	5	3	3	21	3	10	53	100
Highways[a]	14	3	15	–	24	1	11	32	100

TSR: three-wheeled scooter taxi; MTW: motorized two-wheelers; HAPV: human and animal powered vehicles.
[a] Statistical summary of 11 locations, not representative for the whole country (tractor fatalities not included).
Source: reproduced from reference *44*, with the permission of the publisher.

vehicles are involved in a large proportion of road traffic collisions (see Box 2.2). These road users increasingly have to share traffic space with four-wheeled vehicles, such as cars, buses and trucks. Road design and traffic management are generally poor and fail to provide adequate safety in such a mix of traffic. High-income countries did not experience this phase of development, with fast vehicles mixing with vulnerable road users, to such a degree (*50*).

BOX 2.2

Bicycles and bicycle injuries

There are some 800 million bicycles in the world, twice the number that there are cars. In Asia alone, bicycles carry more people than do all the world's cars. Nonetheless, in many countries, bicycle injuries are not given proper recognition as a road safety problem and attract little research (*45*).

In Beijing, China, about a third of all traffic deaths occur among bicyclists (*46*). In India, bicyclists represent between 12% and 21% of road user fatalities, the second-largest category after pedestrians (*47*).

China is one of the few developing countries where public policy until recently has encouraged the use of bicycles as a form of commuting. In the city of Tianjin, 77% of all daily passenger trips are taken by bicycle – compared, for instance, with just 1% in Sydney, Australia (*48*). There are estimated to be over 300 million bicycles in all of China. While about one in four people in China owns a bicycle, only 1 in 74 000 owns a car (*45*). Use of bicycle helmets in China is rare, though. In the city of Wuhan, for instance, their use is non-existent, despite the fact that 45% of all traffic deaths in the city occur among bicyclists (*49*).

Reducing bicycle injuries

To reduce bicycle injuries – in China, as elsewhere – several types of intervention are likely to be effective.
Changes to the road environment can be highly beneficial. They include:
— separating bicycles from other forms of traffic;
— engineering measures to control traffic flow and reinforce low speeds;
— bicycle lanes;
— traffic signals and signs aimed at bicyclists;
— painted lines on the side of the road;
— removing obstacles from roads and cycle paths;
— creating clear lines of sight;
— repairing road surfaces, to remove pot-holes and dangerous curbs.
Measures involving changes in personal behaviour include:
— use of a bicycle helmet;
— safe bicycling practices;
— respectful behaviour towards others sharing the road.

BOX 2.2 (continued)

Legislative and related measures that can be effective include:
   laws mandating helmet use;
   strict legal limits on alcohol use while bicycling;
   speed restrictions;
   enforcement of traffic laws.

Introducing a package of all these approaches is likely to be more effective than if they are used singly, and promises in all countries to significantly reduce the toll of bicycle-related injuries.

Occupational road traffic injuries

Motor vehicle crashes are the leading cause of death in the workplace in the United States, and contribute substantially to the road fatality burden in other industrialized nations. In the United States, an average of 2100 workers died from motor vehicle crashes each year between 1992 and 2001, accounting for 35% of all workplace fatalities in that country, and representing slightly over 3% of the total road crash fatalities (S. Pratt, personal communication, 2003) (*51*).

In the European Union, road traffic and transport crashes at work account for an even greater proportion of workplace fatalities – around 41% in 1999 (*52*). In Australia, the experience is similar, with nearly half of all workplace fatalities between 1989 and 1992 associated with either driving for work or commuting between home and the workplace. Work-related crashes were estimated to comprise 13% of all road fatalities (*53*). Data for Australia, however, differ from those for the European Union and the United States in that work-related crashes include those that occur during commuting to and from work in addition to driving during the workday. Data on work-related road traffic crashes in low-income and middle-income countries are scant.

Sex and age

The distribution of road traffic mortality rates by sex and age, globally, as well as for each WHO region, is shown in the Statistical Annex, Table A.2. Over 50% of the global mortality due to road traffic injury occurs among young adults aged between 15 and 44 years (*54*), and the rates for this age group are higher in low-income and middle-income countries. In 2002, males accounted for 73% of all road traffic deaths, with an overall rate almost three times that for females: 27.6 per 100 000 population and 10.4 per 100 000 population, respectively. Road traffic mortality rates are higher in men than in women in all regions regardless of income level, and also across all age groups (Figure 2.8). On average, males in the low-income and middle-income countries of the WHO Africa Region and the WHO Eastern Mediterranean Region have the highest road traffic injury mortality rates worldwide (see Statistical Annex, Table A.2). The gender difference in mortality rates is probably related to both exposure and risk-taking behaviour.

Table 2.7 shows the burden of road traffic injuries in terms of DALYs by sex. Morbidity rates for males are considerably higher than those for females. Furthermore, about 60% of the DALYs lost globally as a result of road traffic injury occurs among adults aged between 15 and 44 years (*54*).

TABLE 2.7

Road traffic injury burden (DALYs lost) by WHO region and sex, 2002			
WHO region	Males	Females	Total
All	27 057 385	11 368 958	38 426 342
African Region	4 665 446	2 392 812	7 058 257
Region of the Americas	3 109 183	1 141 861	4 251 044
South-East Asia Region	7 174 901	2 856 994	10 031 894
European Region	2 672 506	937 945	3 610 451
Eastern Mediterranean Region	3 173 548	1 403 037	4 576 585
Western Pacific Region	6 261 800	2 636 309	8 898 110

DALYs: Disability-adjusted life years.

Source: WHO Global Burden of Disease project, 2002, Version 1 (see Statistical Annex).

FIGURE 2.8

Road traffic deaths by sex and age group, world, 2002

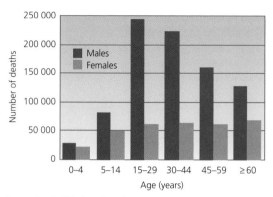

Source: WHO Global Burden of Disease project, 2002, Version 1 (see Statistical Annex).

As expected, when analysed by country, road traffic injury mortality rates are again substantially higher among males than among females. El Salvador's road traffic fatality rate for males, for instance, is 58.1 per 100 000, compared with 13.6 per 100 000 for females (see Statistical Annex, Table A.4). In Latvia, there is a similar gender difference, with a rate of 42.7 per 100 000 for men and 11.4 per 100 000 for females. Certain factors in some countries give rise to an even greater gap between the genders; females may be excluded as drivers or passengers, and in general may face less exposure to road traffic crash risk for cultural or economic reasons.

A comprehensive review of 46 studies in low-income and middle-income countries found that, in terms of involvement in road traffic crashes, there was a consistent predominance of males over females; males were involved in a mean of 80% of crashes, and 87% of drivers were male (30). Recent studies from China, Colombia, Ghana, Kenya, Mexico, Mozambique, the Republic of Korea, Thailand, Trinidad and Tobago, Viet Nam and Zambia all indicate greater rates of male as opposed to female involvement in road traffic collisions (55).

According to WHO data, adults aged between 15 and 44 years account for more than 50% of all road traffic deaths. In high-income countries, adults aged between 15 and 29 years have the highest rates of injury, while in low-income and middle-income countries rates are highest among those over the age of 60 years (see Statistical Annex, Table A.2).

Of all the age groups, children under 15 years of age have the lowest mortality rates (both sexes), due in large measure to the lower rate of exposure they experience (see Statistical Annex, Table A.2 and Box 2.3). These rates vary by region – the WHO African Region and the WHO Eastern Mediterranean Region both show fatality rates of above 18 per 100 000 for male children under the age of 15 years. Globally, the road traffic fatality rate for male children aged 5 to 14 years is slightly higher than that for female children (13.2 per 100 000, against 8.2 per 100 000).

BOX 2.3
Children and road traffic injury

Child road trauma is a major worldwide problem. Children are especially vulnerable, as their physical and cognitive skills are not fully developed and their smaller stature makes it hard for them to see and to be seen. Societies are concerned about the basic safety of their children.

Road trauma is a leading cause of injury to children. In high-income countries, child injury and road deaths rose sharply with motorization in the 1950s and 1960s. While many of these countries have had great success in prevention, road traffic crashes remain a leading cause of death and injury for children. In low-income and middle-income countries, child deaths and injuries are rising as the number of vehicles increases.

According to WHO estimates for 2002, there were 180 500 children killed as the result of road crashes. Some 97% of these child road deaths occurred in low-income and middle-income countries.

The level and pattern of child road injury is linked to differences in road use. In Africa, children are more likely to be hurt as pedestrians and as users of public transport. In south-east Asia, it is as pedestrians, bicyclists and, increasingly, as passengers on motor scooters, and in Europe and North America, it is as passengers in private motor cars and as pedestrians that children are at greatest risk of a road traffic injury.

BOX 2.3 (continued)

The burden of injury is unequal. More boys are injured than girls, and children from poorer families have higher rates of injury. Even in high-income countries, research has shown that children from poorer families and ethnic minority groups have higher rates of unintentional injury, particularly in the case of child pedestrians.

Many countries have made substantial improvements in child road safety. In Australia, for example, in the 25 years after 1970, the road fatality rate per 100 000 children fell by 60% (56).

Interventions that have done much to reduce child traffic injuries and deaths include:

— the development, promotion and increasing use of specifically-designed child restraints;
— improvements in the road environment that have reduced the number of child pedestrian injuries, since these injuries are associated with traffic volume and traffic speed (57);
— increased use of bicycle helmets, that has been associated with a reduction in head injuries among children.

The success, though, of prevention efforts in child road injury is not uniform, and much remains to be done. As noted by Deal et al. (58), "Injuries, both violent and intentional, are one of the most significant public health issues facing children today, but public outrage is absent. As a result, proven solutions go unused, and thousands of children die each year."

Around the world, 193 478 older persons (aged 60 years and above) died in 2002 as a result of road traffic crashes; this figure is equivalent to 16% of the global total (see Statistical Annex, Table A.2 and Box 2.4).

In some countries, the over-60 years age group accounts for a higher proportion of all road traffic deaths than the global average. A study conducted in 1998 in the United Kingdom found that 25.4% of all road traffic fatalities were people aged 60 years or above. In terms of distribution by road user group, 46.6% of pedestrian fatalities and 53% of bus passenger fatalities were people aged 60 years and above. Except for bicyclists, this age group was overrepresented in all categories of road traffic fatalities (61). The OECD (62) found that in 1997, pedestrian fatalities among those aged 65 years and above were lowest in the Netherlands (5.5% of all road traffic fatalities) and highest in Norway (49%) and the United Kingdom (48.8%).

Qatar and the United Arab Emirates both display high mortality rates among the over-60 years age group. In Qatar, males over 60 years had a road traffic fatality rate more than twice that of those in the 15–29 years age group (110 per 100 000, against 48 per 100 000) (63). In the United Arab Emirates, the rates were lower but the difference between age groups was more marked: 29 per 100 000 for those aged 15–44 years and 91 per 100 000 for those aged 60 years or above (64).

No specific studies on older persons and road traffic injuries in low-income and middle-income countries could be found. However, results of a study on adult pedestrian traffic trauma in Cape Town, South Africa, found that only 18% of persons involved in collisions were aged 60 years or above (65).

Socioeconomic status and location

Socioeconomic status is well known to be a risk factor for injury generally, and road traffic injury is no exception (10, 42, 66–68). Studies have found that individuals from disadvantaged socioeconomic groups or living in poorer areas are at greatest risk of being killed or injured as a result of a road traffic crash, even in high-income countries. The evidence suggests that explanations for these differences should be sought in variations in exposure to risk, rather than in behaviour (67), though behavioural differences do play some role. Even in industrialized countries, road traffic injuries as a cause of mortality have the steepest social class gradient, particularly in the case of children and young adults (67, 69).

There are several indicators that are widely used to assess socioeconomic status, educational and occupational level being two of the most common. In a New Zealand cohort study conducted in the 1990s, it was found that drivers with low-status occupations and lower levels of education had a higher risk of injury, even when adjusting for confounding variables such as driving exposure levels (70). In Sweden, the risk of injury for pedestrians and bicyclists was between 20% and 30% higher among the children of manual workers than those of higher-salaried employees (67).

BOX 2.4

Older people and road traffic injury

From a public health point of view, the most serious problem facing the elderly relates to the fact that their mobility out of doors may be restricted because the transport system has failed to meet their needs. Safety issues tend to be a secondary issue.

Road traffic injuries are not a major cause of death for the elderly. However, relative to their proportion of the overall population, older people are often overrepresented in traffic fatalities, especially as vulnerable road users. Older pedestrians in particular are associated with a very high rate of road injury and death. This is mainly due to the increased physical frailty of the elderly. Given the same type of impact, an older person is more likely to be injured or killed than a younger one.

Because of the mobility it provides, private car travel can be more important for the elderly than for those in other age groups. Many people continue to drive vehicles until they are very old. For some, driving may be their only option for mobility, since certain illnesses can affect their ability to walk or to use public transport before affecting their ability to drive.

There is a widespread misconception that older drivers are a threat to traffic safety. Generally speaking, older drivers have the lowest crash rates of all age groups, but because of their frailty, have higher injury and fatality rates (59, 60). Their injury rates may also be affected by diseases such as osteoporosis, impaired homeostasis and poor tissue elasticity.

Older drivers face different types of crashes than younger ones. They experience relatively more crashes in complex traffic situations, such as at intersections, and relatively fewer through lack of caution, such as through speeding or careless overtaking. Injury patterns also differ, partly because of differences in the nature of collisions, with older people suffering more fatal chest injuries, for instance, than younger drivers.

Recent studies on ageing and transport have highlighted pedestrian safety as the main safety concern for the elderly. These studies have indicated that if good quality door-to-door public transport is not available for the elderly, then the use of private cars remains their safest option for getting around. While it is accepted that certain groups of older drivers should not drive – such as those suffering from advanced forms of dementia – mandatory screening of drivers based on age is not recommended. Improvements in pedestrian infrastructure, and interventions to support safe driving as long as possible for older people, are generally regarded as better investments for their safety and mobility than attempts to stop them from driving.

The choice of transport in developing countries is often influenced by socioeconomic factors, especially income. In Kenya, for example, 27% of commuters who had had no formal education were found to travel on foot, 55% used buses or mini-buses and 8% travelled in private cars. By contrast, 81% of those with secondary-level education usually travelled in private cars, 19% by bus and none walked (43).

In many countries, road traffic crashes are more frequent in urban areas, particularly as urbanization increases. However, injury severity is generally greater in rural areas. This could be related to road design and congestion in urban areas slowing traffic, while conditions in rural areas allow for travelling at greater speeds. In low-income and middle-income countries, fewer crashes happen in rural areas, but the overall costs to the families can be greater when they do occur (71). In many countries there is concern over the vulnerability of people living along highways, since these roads are often built through areas where economic activity already exists, thus creating potential conflicts over space between the road users and the local population (55).

Other health, social and economic impacts

Estimating the cost to society of road crashes is important for several reasons. First, it is essential for raising awareness of the seriousness of road crashes as a social problem, Second, it serves to make proper comparisons between road traffic crashes and other causes of death and injury. Third, since the social cost of road traffic crashes is a reflection of the social benefits of reducing crashes through safety interventions, scientific assessments of the costs enables priorities between different interventions to be made, using cost–benefit methods.

Assessment of road traffic injury costs can be carried out with methods that are well known in the health valuation literature. Though the costs to society – such as lost productivity and economic opportunity, and diverted institutional resources – can be estimated in economic terms, valuing the suffering and loss of life associated with road traffic injuries is difficult and often contentious. Accordingly, some studies measure what people would pay – referred to as their "willingness to pay"– to reduce the risk of a fatal or non-fatal injury. Another method is to equate the loss of life through traffic crashes with lost earnings. This is known as the "human capital" approach. In any case, the social cost of an injury or premature death should at least include the associated costs of medical treatment – the direct costs of illness – as well as the loss in productivity associated with the death or injury – the indirect costs of illness. The costs of medical treatment normally include emergency treatment, initial medical costs, and, for serious injuries, the costs of long-term care and rehabilitation. Productivity losses include the value of lost household services and the value of lost earnings for the victim, caregivers and family. In practice, many analyses of the costs of traffic crashes, especially those in developing countries, use lost productivity, rather than willingness-to-pay, to value injury and death.

Industrialized countries regularly produce annual estimates of the overall cost of road traffic crashes. These estimates include the cost of injuries and fatalities sustained in crashes and the cost of damage to property, as well as administrative costs associated with crashes, such as legal expenses and the costs of administering insurance, and the value of the delays in travel caused by crashes. Of all of these costs, those of injuries and fatalities are perhaps the most difficult to value. Medical and rehabilitation costs can be prohibitively expensive and often continue for an indefinite time, particularly in the case of serious road traffic disabilities. Though most attention is usually focused on fatalities, injuries and their ensuing disabilities take an unexpectedly costly toll.

Some major gaps exist in the research on the health and socioeconomic impacts of road traffic injuries. First, existing analyses of costs do not address particularly well those costs related to psychosocial issues, such as pain and suffering. Second, there is a lack of good international standards for predicting and measuring disability. In addition, there are far fewer studies of the cost of traffic crashes in developing countries than elsewhere. One reason for this is the scarcity of reliable data on the number and nature of crashes.

Health and social impacts

Injuries sustained by victims of a road traffic crash vary in type and severity. Data from the GBD 2002 project show that almost a quarter of those injured severely enough to require admission to a health facility sustain a traumatic brain injury; 10% suffer open wounds, such as lacerations, and nearly 20% experience fractures to the lower limbs (see Table 2.8). Studies in both developed and developing countries have found that motor vehicle crashes are the leading cause of traumatic brain injury (65, 72–76).

A review of studies in low-income and middle-income countries (30) revealed that road traffic-related injury accounted for between 30% and 86% of trauma admissions in these countries. Eleven of the 15 studies that included data on hospital utilization examined the length of stay. The overall mean length of stay was 20 days, ranging from 3.8 days in Jordan to 44.6 days in Sharjah, United Arab Emirates. Patients who sustained spinal injury had the longest duration of hospital stay.

The review further found the following:
- Road traffic injury patients comprised between 13% and 31% of all injury-related attendees in hospitals.
- Road traffic injury patients represented 48% of bed occupancy in surgical wards in some countries.
- Road traffic injury patients were the most frequent users of operating theatres and intensive care units.

TABLE 2.8

The 20 leading non-fatal injuries sustained[a] as a result of road traffic collisions, world, 2002

Type of injury sustained	Rate per 100 000 population	Proportion of all traffic injuries
Intracranial injury[b] (short-term[c])	85.3	24.6
Open wound	35.6	10.3
Fractured patella, tibia or fibula	26.9	7.8
Fractured femur (short-term[c])	26.1	7.5
Internal injuries	21.9	6.3
Fractured ulna or radius	19.2	5.5
Fractured clavicle, scapula or humerus	16.7	4.8
Fractured facial bones	11.4	3.3
Fractured rib or sternum	11.1	3.2
Fractured ankle	10.8	3.1
Fractured vertebral column	9.4	2.7
Fractured pelvis	8.8	2.6
Sprains	8.3	2.4
Fractured skull (short-term[c])	7.9	2.3
Fractured foot bones	7.2	2.1
Fractured hand bones	6.8	2.0
Spinal cord injury (long-term[d])	4.9	1.4
Fractured femur (long-term[d])	4.3	1.3
Intracranial injury[b] (long-term[d])	4.3	1.2
Other dislocation	3.4	1.0

[a] Requiring admission to a health facility.
[b] Traumatic brain injury.
[c] Short-term = lasts only a matter of weeks.
[d] Long-term = lasts until death, with some complications resulting in reduced life expectancy.
Source: WHO Global Burden of Disease project, 2002, Version 1.

- Increased workloads in X-ray departments and increased demands for physiotherapy and rehabilitation services were, to a large extent, attributable to road traffic crashes.

Individual country studies report similar findings. For instance, out of a total of 2913 trauma patients who had attended the University of Ilorin teaching hospital in Nigeria over a period of 15 months, 1816, or 62.3%, had suffered road traffic injuries (77). In Kenya, a survey on the perceived capacity of health care facilities to handle more than 10 injured persons simultaneously, showed that only 40% of health administrators thought that their facilities were well prepared. Of the hospitals that were least prepared, 74% were public hospitals – the facilities that poor people use most frequently (43).

The results of a study in the United States (78) revealed that 5.27 million people had sustained non-fatal road traffic injuries in 2000, 87% of which were considered "minor", according to the maximum injury severity scale. These injuries resulted in medical costs of US$ 31.7 billion, placing a huge burden on health care services and individual finances. In terms of unit medical costs per injury level, the most severe level of injury – MAIS 5, that includes head and spinal cord injury – cost by far the largest amount, at US$ 332 457 per injury, exceeding the combined cost per unit of all other injuries, including fatalities.

Injured people often suffer physical pain and emotional anguish that is beyond any economic compensation. Permanent disability, such as paraplegia, quadriplegia, loss of eyesight, or brain damage, can deprive an individual of the ability to achieve even minor goals and result in dependence on others for economic support and routine physical care. Less serious – but more common – injuries to ankles, knees and the cervical spine can result in chronic physical pain and limit an injured person's physical activity for lengthy periods. Serious burns, contusions and lacerations can lead to emotional trauma associated with permanent disfigurement (79).

Psychosocial impact

Medical costs and lost productivity do not capture the psychosocial losses associated with road traffic crashes, either to those injured or to their families. These costs might possibly exceed the productivity losses and medical costs associated with premature death, were they accurately quantifiable. A study conducted in Sweden showed that there was a high rate of psychosocial complications following road traffic crashes, even for minor injuries. Almost half the respondents in the study group still reported travel anxiety two years after the crash. Pain, fear and fatigue were also commonly found. Of those employed, 16% could not return to their ordinary jobs, while a third reported a reduction in leisure-time activities (*80*).

Road traffic crashes can place a heavy burden on the family and friends of the injured person, many of whom also experience adverse social, physical and psychological effects, in the short-term or long-term. In the European Union, more than 40 000 people are killed and more than 150 000 disabled for life by road traffic crashes each year. As a result, nearly 200 000 families annually are newly bereaved or have family members disabled for life (*81*). In a study on how families and communities cope with injured relatives, the most frequently reported coping strategy was reallocation of work within the family, with at least one family member having to take time off from their usual activity to help the injured person or to carry on that person's work. As a result of individuals changing their work patterns for this reason, about a third of them lost income. In some cases, the injury of a family member caused children to stay away from school (*82*).

The Fédération Européenne des Victimes de la Route (FEVR) conducted a comprehensive study in Europe of the physical, psychological and material damage suffered by victims and their families subsequent to road crashes (*83*). The results showed that 90% of the families of those killed and 85% of the families of those disabled reported a significant permanent decline in their quality of life, and in half of the cases the consequences were especially severe. In a follow-up study, FEVR sought to determine the causes of this decline. Most of the victims or their relatives suffered from headaches, sleeping problems, disturbing nightmares and general health problems. Three years after the incident, these complaints had not significantly decreased (*84*). In addition, it was found that victims and their families were often dissatisfied with such matters as criminal proceedings, insurance and civil claims, and the level of support and information received on legal rights and other issues (*84*).

The psychological and social consequences of road traffic trauma are not always directly propor-tional to the severity of the physical injury; even relatively minor injuries can have profound psychosocial effects. Nearly a fifth of those injured, according to one study, developed an acute stress reaction and a quarter displayed psychiatric problems within the first year. Long-term psychiatric problems consisted mainly of mood disorder (in around 10% of cases), phobic travel anxiety (20%) and post-traumatic stress disorder (11%). Phobic travel disorder was frequent among drivers and passengers (*85*).

Other consequences

In a recent study, 55% of those attending an accident and emergency unit following a road traffic crash reported significant medical, psychiatric, social or legal consequences one year later. Many patients with less serious or no injuries still suffered long-term health and other problems not necessarily related to their injury. Furthermore, reports of continuing physical problems one year on, largely musculoskeletal in nature, were considerably more common than would be expected from the nature of injuries sustained (*86*).

Pedestrians and motorcyclists suffer the most severe injuries as a result of motor vehicle collisions, report more continuing medical problems and require more assistance, compared with other types of road user. There are few psychological or social differences, however, between different road users (*87*).

In many low-income and middle-income countries, and sometimes in high-income countries as well, the cost of prolonged care, the loss of the primary breadwinner, funeral costs, and the loss of income due to disability, can push a family into poverty (*10, 38*). The process of impoverishment can affect children especially strongly. The second leading cause of orphaned children in Mexico is the loss of parents as a result of road traffic crashes (*38*).

Other consequential effects of transport and motorization on the environment and health are dealt with more comprehensively in recent WHO documents (*88, 89*).

Economic impact

As part of the recent review undertaken by the United Kingdom-based TRL Ltd on the number of road traffic collisions globally, information on road crash costs from 21 developed and developing countries was analysed (2). This study found that the average annual cost of road crashes was about 1% of GNP in developing countries, 1.5% in countries in economic transition and 2% in highly-motorized countries (see Table 2.9). According to this study, the annual burden of economic costs globally is estimated at around US$ 518 billion. On a country basis, the economic burdens are estimated to represent proportions of GNP ranging from 0.3% in Viet Nam to almost 5% in Malawi and in Kwa-Zulu-Natal, South Africa (2), with a few countries registering even higher percentages. In most countries, though, the costs exceed 1% of GNP.

TABLE 2.9

Road crash costs by region

Region[a]	GNP, 1997 (US$ billion)	Estimated annual crash costs	
		As percentage of GNP	Costs (US$ billion)
Africa	370	1	3.7
Asia	2 454	1	24.5
Latin America and Caribbean	1 890	1	18.9
Middle East	495	1.5	7.4
Central and Eastern Europe	659	1.5	9.9
Subtotal	5 615		64.5
Highly-motorized countries[b]	22 665	2	453.3
Total			517.8

GNP: gross national product.

[a] Data are displayed according to the regional classifications of the TRL Ltd, United Kingdom.

[b] Australia, Japan, New Zealand, North America, and the western European countries.

Source: reproduced from reference 2, with minor editorial amendments, with the permission of the author.

The total annual costs of road crashes to low-income and middle-income countries are estimated to be about US$ 65 billion, exceeding the total annual amount received in development assistance (2). These costs are especially damaging for countries struggling with the problems of development. In the high-income countries of the European Union, it has been estimated that the cost of road crashes each year exceeds €180 billion – twice the European Union annual budget for all of its activities (90, 91).

A study carried out in the United States, using the human capital – or lost productivity – approach, estimated the national economic costs of road traffic crashes at US$ 230.6 billion, or 2.3% of GDP (78).

Research in Australia put that country's economic costs at 3.6% of GDP (92). The cost of traffic crashes as a proportion of GDP for other high-income countries, calculated using the human capital approach, ranges from 0.5% for Great Britain (1990) and 0.9% for Sweden (1995) to 2.8% for Italy (1997) (93). Averaging the cost of traffic crashes in the 1990s across 11 high-income countries, gives an average cost equivalent to 1.4% of GDP (93).

Information on costs from low-income and middle-income countries is generally scant. A recent study from Bangladesh, comparing data from a household survey with official police reports, suggests that the police record about one-third of all traffic fatalities and 2% of serious injuries (94). When adjustments were made for this level of underreporting, the cost of traffic crashes in Bangladesh in 2000 was estimated at Tk38 billion (US$ 745 million) or about 1.6% of GDP.

The cost of road traffic collisions in South Africa for 2000 were estimated at approximately R13.8 billion (US$ 2 billion) (95). On the assumption that 80% of seriously-injured and 50% of slightly-injured road traffic collision victims would seek care at a state hospital, basic hospital costs alone for the first year of treatment were calculated to cost the government of the order of R321 million (US$ 46.4 million) (96).

Uganda has an annual road traffic fatality rate of 160 deaths per 10 000 vehicles, one of the highest in Africa. Based on average damage costs per vehicle of US$ 2290, an average fatality cost of US$ 8600 and average injury costs of US$ 1933, road traffic collisions cost the Ugandan economy around US$ 101 million per year, representing 2.3% of the country's GNP (97). In the mid-1990s, the cost of road traffic injuries in Côte d'Ivoire was estimated to be 1% of GNP (98).

Eastern Europe does not fare much better. The estimated economic costs of motor vehicle traffic incidents in 1998 were in the range US$ 66.6 – 80.6 million for Estonia, US$ 162.7 – 194.7 million for Latvia, and US$ 230.5 – 267.5 million for Lithuania. The majority of these costs are related to injury, in which the loss of market and household productivity and the cost of medical care predominate. Property damage represents around 16% of the total for Estonia and 17% for Latvia and Lithuania (79).

Using the notion of, "potentially productive years of life lost", injuries in 1999 cost China 12.6 million years, more than any other disease group. The estimated annual economic cost of injury in China is equivalent to US$ 12.5 billion – almost four times the total public health services budget for the country and a productivity loss that more than offsets the total productivity gains of new entrants to the labour force each year. Motor vehicle fatalities alone accounted for 25% of the total number of potentially productive years of life lost from all injury deaths, with their potential impact on economic development being particularly acute in rural areas (99).

The most productive age group, those aged between 15 and 44 years, is heavily represented in road traffic injuries; the economic impacts of injuries in this age group are therefore especially damaging. According to WHO, injuries to individuals in this age group, "tend to affect productivity severely, particularly among the lowest-income groups whose exposure to risk is greatest and whose earning capacity is most likely to rely on physical activity" (100). The incidence of road traffic crashes in Kenya illustrates this point; more than 75% of road traffic casualties are among economically productive young adults (30).

A case study conducted in Bangladesh found that poor families were more likely than those better off to lose their head of household and thus suffer immediate economic effects as a result of road traffic injuries. The loss of earnings, together with medical bills, funeral costs and legal bills, can have a ruinous effect on a family's finances. Among the poor, 32% of the road deaths surveyed occurred to a head of household or that head's spouse, compared with 21% among those not defined as poor. Over 70% of households reported that their household income, food consumption and food production had decreased after a road death. Three quarters of all poor households affected by a road death reported a decrease in their living standard, compared with 58% of other households. In addition, 61% of poor families had to borrow money as a result of a death, compared with 34% of other families (94).

In cases where there is prolonged treatment or the death of the victim, the family may end up selling most of its assets, including land, and possibly becoming trapped in long-term indebtedness (82).

Data and evidence for road traffic injury prevention

Two of the central aims of modern medicine are to advance knowledge and promote practices that are based on evidence. This emphasis on evidence reflects the need to continuously review and strengthen the evidence base for public health interventions. This applies not only to communicable diseases but also to noncommunicable diseases and injuries, such as road traffic injuries. This section discusses issues and concerns related to road traffic injury data and evidence.

Why collect data and build evidence on road traffic injuries?

Road safety is of prime concern to many individuals, groups and organizations, all of whom require data and evidence. While different users have different data needs, reliable data and evidence are essential for describing the burden of road traffic injuries, assessing risk factors, developing and evaluating interventions, providing information for policy-makers and decision-makers, and raising awareness. Without reliable information, the priorities for road traffic injury prevention cannot be rationally or satisfactorily determined.

Sources and types of data

Police departments and hospitals provide most of the data used in road traffic injury prevention and road safety. In addition to the sources indicated in Table 2.10, data are also available from published documents, such as journals, books and research reports, as well as on the Internet.

There are a number of approaches to collecting and keeping data and evidence on road traffic injuries. These approaches are well documented, both for injuries in general and road traffic injuries in particular (*101–104*).

Injury surveillance systems

Most countries have some form of national system for aggregating data on road crashes using police records or hospital records, or both. However, the quality and reliability of data vary between surveillance systems in different countries and also between systems within the same country. For road traffic injuries, certain key variables need to be collected. WHO, in its recently

TABLE 2.10

Key sources of road traffic injury data

Source	Type of data	Comments
Police	Number of road traffic incidents, fatalities and injuries Type of road users involved Age and sex of casualties Type of vehicles involved Police assessment of causes of crashes Location and sites of crashes Prosecutions	Level of detail varies from one country to another. Police records can be inaccessible. Underreporting is a common problem, particularly in low-income and middle-income countries.
Health settings (e.g. hospital inpatient records, emergency room records, trauma registries, ambulance or emergency technician records, health clinic records, family doctor records)	Fatal and non-fatal injuries Age and sex of casualties Costs of treatment	Level of detail varies from one health care facility to another. Injury data may be recorded under "other causes", making it difficult to extract for analysis.
Insurance firms	Fatal and non-fatal injuries Damage to vehicles Costs of claims	Access to these data may be difficult.
Other private and public institutions, including transport companies	Number of fatal and non-fatal injuries occurring among employees Damage and losses Insurance claims Legal issues Operational data	These data may be specific to the planning and operation of the firms.
Government departments and specialized agencies collecting data for national planning and development	Population denominators Income and expenditure data Health indicators Exposure data Pollution data Energy consumption Literacy levels	These data are complementary and important for analysis of road traffic injuries. The data are collected by different ministries and organizations, though there may be one central agency that compiles and produces reports, such as statistical abstracts, economic surveys and development plans.
Special interest groups (e.g. research institutes, advocacy nongovernmental organizations, victim support organizations, transport unions, consulting firms, institutions involved in road safety activities)	Number of road traffic incidents, fatal and non-fatal injuries Type of road users involved Age and sex of casualties Type of vehicles involved Causes Location and sites of crashes Social and psychological impacts Interventions	The various organizations have different interests.

published *Injury surveillance guidelines*, makes recommendations for a minimum data set for surveillance of road traffic injuries in emergency rooms (*101*).

Most high-income countries have well established injury surveillance systems. Recently, a number of low-income and middle-income countries have set up systems to monitor injuries, including road traffic injuries. Examples include Colombia (C. Clavel-Arcas, unpublished observations, 2003), El Salvador (C. Clavel-Arcas, unpublished observations, 2003), Ethiopia (*105*), Ghana (*106*), Jamaica (*107*), Mozambique (*105*), Nicaragua (C. Clavel-Arcas, unpublished observations, 2003), South Africa (*108*), Thailand (*109*) and Uganda (*110*) (see Box 2.5).

BOX 2.5
The national injury surveillance system in Thailand

Thailand's provincial injury surveillance system started in 1993. Its objectives were to establish a database to evaluate, at a provincial level, the quality of acute trauma care and the referral services provided to the injured, and to improve injury prevention and control at both local and national levels (*109*). Previously, data providers in hospitals had not been responsible for information on road traffic crashes at a provincial level. Existing information systems were poorly designed and managed, not computerized, and not standardized as regards definitions, sources of data and methods of data collection. Consequently, regional or national comparisons were impossible (*109*).

A trauma registry system had been developed in the large provincial hospital in Khon Kaen. This system was chosen as the prototype for the new surveillance system, because of its achievements over eight years in injury prevention and improving the quality of acute care (*111*). The Noncommunicable Diseases Epidemiology Section of the Ministry of Public Health revised the hospital's trauma registry form and set up appropriate reporting criteria, definitions of terms and methods of coding. Appropriate computer software for processing the data was developed. The hospital produced manuals and ran training courses to help personnel operate the surveillance system effectively (*109*).

In January 1995, a provincial injury surveillance system was established in five sentinel hospitals, one in Bangkok and four in other regions of Thailand. Each was a large general hospital with a sufficient number of injuries and mix of cases, receiving referrals from other local hospitals (*109*).

All those acutely injured within seven days before admittance, including those who had died, were included in the surveillance system. Data were forwarded every six months by the local authorities to the central coordinating unit in the Epidemiology Division of the Ministry of Public Health.

Within six months, it had become clear that traffic injuries were the most important cause of injury in each sentinel hospital. The epidemiology of other major causes of injuries was also investigated, and the quality of pre-hospital service and of inter-hospital transfers was monitored. Information obtained was fed into the eighth five-year National Health Development Plan (*112*).

Data on alcohol-related traffic injuries were instrumental in the introduction of obligatory warnings on the labels of alcoholic beverages and of other interventions against drink-driving. The surveillance reports were sent to policy-makers in a range of sectors, including parliamentarians and governors of the provinces in which the sentinel hospitals were located – as well as to police departments and the mass media (*109, 76*).

Although the extra workload arising from the surveillance activities created problems in the sentinel hospitals, the advantages of the scheme were such that 20 more hospitals voluntarily joined the surveillance network (*76*). Simplifications to the system were subsequently made, though, to reduce the workload on medical records departments, so that the sentinel hospitals were required to report only cases of severe injury, including:
— deaths before arrival;
— deaths in the emergency department;
— observed or admitted injury cases.
This caused only minor changes in ranking among the top five leading causes of injury (*76*).

In January 2001, Thailand's National Injury Surveillance was officially launched. By 2003, the national network had grown to include 28 large hospitals, as well as almost 60 general hospitals and one university hospital. The system is one of only a few injury surveillance systems in low-income and middle-income countries that operate nationally and involve a model that WHO recognizes and encourages for technology transfer between countries.

In addition to country-specific information systems, a number of regional systems exist. Countries belonging to the OECD support and make use of the International Road Traffic Accident Database (IRTAD), to which they submit standardized crash and injury data, together with some basic transport statistics and other safety-related information (13). The United Nations Economic and Social Commission for Asia and the Pacific has developed a regional road crash database known as the Asia-Pacific Road Accident Database (113) which, like IRTAD, requires countries in the region to submit data in a standard format. The Caribbean Epidemiology Centre has introduced an injury surveillance system in the Bahamas, Barbados, and Trinidad and Tobago (114).

Europe has its own regional system, known as CARE – Community Database on Accidents on the Roads in Europe – which differs from the above-mentioned systems in that country returns are mandatory. However, the system allows countries to make returns in their own national formats and it includes disaggregated data on individual crashes. After being received, the data are adjusted for variations in definitions. To this end, a number of correction factors have been developed (115).

International and regional guidelines are available on crash and injury information systems to help countries decide on which data to collect. For example, in the transport sector, the Association of South East Asia Nations has developed road safety guidelines that include advice on what information is required (116). The WHO guidelines for developing and implementing injury surveillance systems in hospital settings contain recommendations on the core minimum data set and supplementary data that should be collected on all injury patients, including road traffic casualties (101).

Community-based surveys

A second approach to gathering data on road traffic injuries is to conduct community-based surveys. Some injured patients fail to reach hospital for a variety of reasons, in which case they will not be captured by hospital-based injury surveillance systems. Community-based surveys not only pick up these otherwise unreported cases, but also provide useful information on injuries and may be of particular relevance in countries where basic population and mortality data are not available (102). Community surveys have been recently conducted in Ghana (117), India (118), Pakistan (119), South Africa (120), Uganda (121) and Viet Nam (122). These surveys, though, require methodological expertise which may not be widely available. To this end, WHO is currently developing *Guidelines for conducting community surveys on injuries and violence*, which will provide a standardized methodology for carrying out such studies (102).

Surveys on selected themes

A third approach is to conduct surveys on particular themes related to road traffic injuries and transport. Examples are road user surveys, road-side surveys, origin–destination surveys, pedestrian surveys, cyclist surveys and speed surveys – as well as studies on such issues as alcohol use and the cost of crashes. These surveys may arise from the need for specific data that are not available from hospital-based surveillance systems or community surveys.

Data linkages

As shown in Table 2.10, road traffic injury data and evidence is collected and stored by a range of agencies. This is in itself a positive feature, as it reflects the multisectoral nature of the phenomenon. However, it also raises important issues to do with access, harmonization and linkages between different data sources and users. Ideally, where there are a number of data sources available, it is important that the data should be linked, to obtain maximum value from the information (see Box 2.6). However, for many countries, especially those with a number of systems at the local level, this is not always the case. A major problem is coordination and sharing of information among different users. While there are usually issues of confidentiality and other legal restrictions involved, it should still be possible to find ways of summarizing the relevant information and making it available, without violating any legal prohibitions.

BOX 2.6

Multidisciplinary crash investigation

An example of in-depth multidisciplinary crash investigation is the Finnish national system, steered and supervised by the Ministry of Transport and Communications and maintained by the Motor Insurers' Centre and the Motor Traffic Insurers Committee (VALT).

The Centre started in-depth crash investigation in 1968 and its 21 law-based investigation teams investigate about 500, mainly fatal crashes, at the scene of the crash, annually. Each team consists of police, a road safety engineer, a vehicle inspector, a medical doctor and sometimes a psychologist. Specific information is collected by each person and a combined report is produced on each case. In each case, more than 500 variables are collected on standardized forms. The emphasis is placed on data that will contribute to crash avoidance and injury prevention. In addition, the teams have legal rights to access information from official and private records and health care systems to obtain human, vehicle and road information.

Coordinated data management systems do exist in a handful of countries. One such example is the United States National Automotive Sampling System, that combines information from four data systems – the Fatality Analysis Reporting System, the General Estimates System, the Crashworthiness Data System and the Crash Injury Research and Engineering Network – to provide an overall picture for policy-makers and decision-makers at the national level (*123*).

For the regular monitoring of road traffic injuries, a system that integrated information from both police sources and health care sources would be ideal. Although there have been a number of pilot projects, such as the one combining police data on fatal crashes with the Hospital In-Patients Statistics database in Scotland (*124*), few countries have established such linked systems on a routine basis.

Analysis of data

Analysing data, producing regular outputs and disseminating information on road traffic injuries are all vital activities. For the purposes of data analysis, there are some excellent software packages available. These systems can build automatic validity checks and quality control into the data management process. Software packages also provide powerful analysis features for diagnosing problems that enable rational decisions to be made on priorities for intervention (*125*).

High standards in data quality assurance and analysis alone are not enough. Road traffic injury information systems also need to allow all appropriate outside bodies access and to ensure that the information is effectively distributed. The design of databases should therefore take account of the principal needs of all their users, providing quality data without overburdening those collecting the data. Databases also require sufficient resources to ensure their sustainability. Countries should collaborate and help support regional and global systems so that the monitoring and evaluation of road safety can be improved and sustained.

Data issues and concerns
Indicators

Indicators are important tools not just for measuring the magnitude of a problem but also for setting targets and assessing performance. The most frequently used absolute and relative indicators for measuring the magnitude of the road traffic injury problem are presented in Table 2.11.

Two very common indicators are the number of deaths per 100 000 population, and the number of deaths per 10 000 vehicles. Both of these indicators have limitations regarding their reliability and validity that place restrictions on how they can be used and interpreted. The number of deaths per 100 000 population is widely used with reasonable confidence to monitor changes over time in "personal risk" levels and to make comparisons between countries. Errors in population statistics are assumed to have little impact on the observed changes or comparisons.

The use of vehicle registrations as an estimate of motorization is also problematical as there can

TABLE 2.11

Examples of commonly used indicators of the road traffic injury problem

Indicator	Description	Use and limitations
Number of injuries	Absolute figure indicating the number of people injured in road traffic crashes	Useful for planning at the local level for emergency medical services
	Injuries sustained may be serious or slight	Useful for calculating the cost of medical care
		Not very useful for making comparisons
		A large proportion of slight injuries are not reported
Number of deaths	Absolute figure indicating the number of people who die as a result of a road traffic crash	Gives a partial estimate of the magnitude of the road traffic problem, in terms of deaths
		Useful for planning at the local level for emergency medical services
		Not very useful for making comparisons
Fatalities per 10 000 vehicles	Relative figure showing ratio of fatalities to motor vehicles	Shows the relationship between fatalities and motor vehicles
		A limited measure of travel exposure because it omits non-motorized transport and other indicators of exposure
Fatalities per 100 000 population	Relative figure showing ratio of fatalities to population	Shows the impact of road traffic crashes on human population
		Useful for estimating severity of crashes
Fatalities per vehicle-kilometre travelled	Number of road deaths per billion kilometres travelled	Useful for international comparisons
		Does not take into account non-motorized travel
Disability-adjusted life years (DALYs)	Measures healthy life years lost due to disability and mortality	DALYs combine both mortality and disability
	One disability-adjusted life year (DALY) lost is equal to one year of healthy life lost, either due to premature death or disability	DALYs do not include all the health consequences associated with injury, such as mental health consequences

be errors in country databases due to delays in adding or removing records of vehicles. Furthermore, changes in vehicle numbers do not generally provide a good estimate of changes in exposure to, and travel on, the road network, especially when making comparisons between countries. A better indicator of traffic safety risk is deaths per vehicle-kilometres, but this also fails to allow for non-motorized travel.

The measurement of exposure to the risk of road traffic injuries presents conceptual and methodological difficulties (*127*). An example of the use of two indicators – fatalities per 100 000 population and fatalities per 10 000 vehicles – is presented in

Figure 2.9. The figure shows that since 1975 Malaysia has experienced a continuous decline in deaths per 10 000 vehicles, whereas the rate of deaths per 100 000 population has shown a slight increase. Over the same period, there has been a rapid growth in motorization and increased mobility among Malaysia's population. The opposing trends in the two indicators reflect the fact that road traffic fatalities have increased more slowly in Malaysia than the growth in the vehicle fleet, but that they have increased a little faster in recent years than the growth in the population. More information is needed to understand how changes in mobility and safety standards have contributed to such trends.

FIGURE 2.9

Road traffic deaths in Malaysia

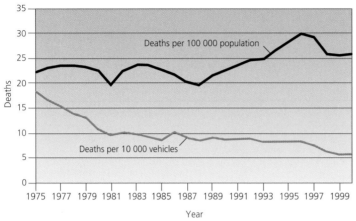

Source: reference *126*.

The relationships between road traffic injuries, motorization and other major risk factors are discussed in more detail in the next chapter.

Though road traffic injury statistics are used as measures of road safety, they are often inadequate and may even be misleading. This highlights the need for existing measures to be refined and new ones to be explored.

Definitions and standardization of data

There are a number of potential problems with the definitions of a road traffic death or injury, arising from:

— variations in the interpretation of the specified time period between the injury event and death;

— the actual interpretation of the definition in different countries and by different people recording the information;

— differing levels of enforcement of definitions;

— differing techniques for assessing the severity of injuries.

The most commonly cited definition of a road traffic fatality is: "any person killed immediately or dying within 30 days as a result of an injury accident" (*128*). However, a recent study has revealed considerable variations in working definitions. For example, in the European Union, Greece, Portugal and Spain use 24 hours, France uses 6 days, Italy uses 7 days and the other countries use 30 days (*129*). To adjust for this

variation, various correction factors are applied to arrive at a 30-day equivalent. Such factors, though, themselves introduce uncertainty as to what the real numbers would be at 30 days.

There are a number of other definitional issues relating to the classification of an injury death as one caused by a road traffic crash, including (*14, 129*):

— the method of assessment;

— the location of a fatal crash (i.e. whether on a public or private road);

— the mode of transport (some classifications stipulate the presence of at least one moving vehicle);

— the source reporting the data (i.e. whether police or a self-report);

— whether or not to include confirmed suicides;

— whether or not post-mortem examinations are routinely conducted on road traffic deaths.

Definitional issues also arise with regard to survivors of road traffic crashes, including:

— the actual definition and interpretation of a serious injury in different countries;

— whether the police, who record most of the information, are sufficiently trained to ascertain and correctly assign injury severity.

In Finland, for example, a serious road traffic injury is considered to involve hospital admission or three days off work; in Sweden, it involves hospital admission as well as fractures, whether or not the patient is admitted; while in France, it involves a hospital stay of at least six days (*129*).

Road traffic injury and death cases can be missed by the data collection system because of differences in the definitions used in different countries and contexts. This issue highlights the need for the standardization of definitions and their application across different countries and settings.

Underreporting

It is clear from studies that underreporting of both deaths and injuries is a major global problem affecting not only low-income and middle-income countries but also high-income ones (*30, 129–131*). In the United Kingdom, studies comparing hospital and police records suggest that some 36% of road traffic injury casualties are not reported to the police (*129*). In addition, around 20% of incidents reported to the police remain unrecorded. In some low-income and middle-income countries, levels of underreporting can be as high as 50% (*2, 132*). Underreporting can arise out of:

— a failure on the part of the public to report;
— the police not recording cases reported to them;
— hospitals not reporting cases presenting to them;
— an exemption for certain institutions, such as the military, from reporting directly to the police.

In some low-income and middle-income countries, underreporting may stem from the basic fact that some victims cannot afford to attend hospital (*133, 134*).

The problem of underreporting highlights a number of structural, methodological and practical issues affecting the quality of data collected on road traffic injuries, including:

— the coordination and reconciliation of data between sources;
— the harmonization and application of agreed definitions, especially the definition of a road crash fatality;
— the actual process of classification and the completion of data forms.

These problems make it difficult to obtain reliable estimates on road traffic fatalities and injuries worldwide and also for certain countries. Harmonization of data at the national and international levels can be facilitated by adopting international definitions. The International Classification of Diseases (ICD-10) (*135*) and the Abbreviated Injury Scale (AIS) can be used for non-fatal road crash injuries (*136*). Agreements to adhere to regional systems such as IRTAD and the Asia-Pacific Road Accident Database will encourage the uniformity of definitions.

Other issues
Studies have uncovered a number of other problems related to road traffic injury data and evidence.

These include:

— missing information within individual records;
— the unavailability of certain specific data (e.g. the crash location, type of injury, identification of the vehicle in which the casualty occurred);
— the scientific soundness of the methods used;
— inadequate quality control;
— lack of data collection on cycling and walking in transport information systems;
— lack of data on exposure;
— the accuracy and completeness of police assessment of cause of crash;
— lack of professionals trained in road safety;
— lack of rigorous evaluation of interventions, particularly in low-income and middle-income countries.

Limitations of the data sources used in this chapter
Although the present assessment of the extent of the burden of road traffic injury is based on the best available global data, it is recognized that the underlying data sources do suffer from a number of limitations. The main ones are outlined below:

• The WHO mortality database lacks complete coverage of vital registration data from all WHO regions. Several countries do not report road traffic incidence data at all. Projected data for some regions are therefore based on relatively small samples of data and can be in error because of missing country information. This has been dealt with by computing estimates using a methodology described in the Statistical Annex. The limitation highlights the need for more countries to submit road traffic injury data to the WHO mortality database.

• The GBD estimates are based largely on 1990 data and although they have been adjusted repeatedly since then, regional and national changes may have made some of the regional projections unreliable. In addition, there is a clear absence of routinely available data, both global and national, on the long-term health and social impacts of road traffic crashes. This shortcoming has led to a reliance on studies undertaken primarily in high-income countries and a corresponding risk of bias if the projected assumptions for low-income and middle-income countries are not accurate.

- The World Bank and TRL Ltd both rely on road traffic mortality data that originated from police sources, and which, in common with WHO data, suffer from problems related to incomplete coverage. There is also the problem of differing definitions of death, that vary from "dead on the spot" to death some time after the crash occurred. The standard definition is "death within 30 days of the crash", though in practice, many countries do not follow it. Both the World Bank and TRL Ltd have made attempts to correct for the underestimates arising from these problems. To correct for different definitions of death, they used the European Conference of Ministers of Transport adjustment for high-income country values (a maximum of 30%, depending on the definition used), and they added 15% to all figures from low-income and middle-income countries (*1, 2*). In addition, both groups made a further correction, adding 2% to the data for high-income countries and 25% for low-income and middle-income countries, to allow for underreporting of road traffic fatalities generally. The TRL study regarded this as a minimum adjustment for underreporting, and set a maximum at +5% for high-income country figures and +50% for low-income and middle-income countries (*2*). The World Bank study base-year data was comparable to the TRL Ltd minimum underreporting data (*1*).

Information on specific topics such as road safety and the elderly, inequality, location (including rural–urban differences), road safety and public transport, and occupational road traffic injuries was extremely limited. Nevertheless, a concerted effort was made to secure all available studies from online databases, published sources and the "grey literature" – such as information published in local, non-indexed journals, government reports and unpublished theses – on these as well as other themes. This yielded a number of studies that have been used to illustrate these topics throughout the chapter.

Conclusion

The problem of road traffic crashes and injuries is growing both in absolute numbers and in relative terms. It is a serious public health and development issue, taxing health care systems and undermining their ability to devote limited resources to other areas of need. The magnitude of road traffic injuries globally can be summarized as follows:

- More than one million people are killed worldwide every year as a result of road traffic crashes.
- Road traffic injuries are the 11th leading cause of death and the 9th leading cause of disability-adjusted life years lost worldwide.
- The poor and vulnerable road users – pedestrians, cyclists and motorcyclists – bear the greatest burden.
- Some 90% of road traffic deaths occur in the developing world, which comprises two thirds of the global population.
- As motorization increases, many low-income and middle-income countries may face a growing toll of road traffic injuries, with potentially devastating consequences in human, social and economic terms.
- Males are more likely to be involved in road traffic crashes than females.
- Economically active adults, aged 15–44 years, account for more than half of all the road traffic deaths.
- Without new or improved interventions, road traffic injuries will be the third leading cause of death by the year 2020.

The health, social and economic impacts of road traffic crashes are substantial.

- Between 20 million and 50 million people sustain an injury as a result of motor vehicle crashes each year.
- Nearly a quarter of all non-fatally injured victims requiring hospitalization sustain a traumatic brain injury as a result of motor vehicle crashes.
- Between 30% and 86% of trauma admissions in some low-income and middle-income countries are the result of road traffic crashes.
- Millions of people are temporarily or permanently disabled as a result of road traffic crashes.

- Many people suffer significant psychological consequences for years following a motor vehicle crash.
- Road traffic crashes cost governments, on average, between 1% and 2% of their gross national product.
- The social costs – more difficult to quantify – exact a heavy toll on victims, their families, friends and communities.
- The death of a breadwinner often pushes a family into poverty.

Accurate data are essential for prioritizing public health issues, monitoring trends and assessing intervention programmes. Many countries have inadequate information systems on road traffic injury, making it difficult to realize the full nature of the problem and thus gain the attention that is required from policy-makers and decision-makers. There are a number of areas where road traffic injury data are often problematic, and these include:

— sources of data (e.g. whether data are from police or health sources);
— the types of data collected;
— inappropriate use of indicators;
— non-standardization of data;
— definitional issues related to traffic deaths and injuries;
— underreporting;
— poor harmonization and linkages between different sources of data.

Governments can help foster stronger collaboration between different groups that collect and keep data and evidence on road traffic injuries. Furthermore, it is essential that data collection and global standards be better coordinated – an area in which the United Nations regional commissions could take a leading role. With such improved collaboration and improved management of data, significant reductions can be achieved in the magnitude of road traffic casualties.

References

1. Kopits E, Cropper M. *Traffic fatalities and economic growth*. Washington, DC, The World Bank, 2003 (Policy Research Working Paper No. 3035).
2. Jacobs G, Aeron-Thomas A, Astrop A. *Estimating global road fatalities*. Crowthorne, Transport Research Laboratory, 2000 (TRL Report 445).
3. *World's first road death*. London, RoadPeace, 2003. (http://www.roadpeace.org/articles/WorldFirstDeath.html, accessed 17 November 2003).
4. Faith N. *Crash: the limits of car safety*. London, Boxtree, 1997.
5. Murray CJL, Lopez AD. *Global health statistics: a compendium of incidence, prevalence and mortality estimates for 200 conditions*. Boston, MA, Harvard School of Public Health, 1996.
6. McGee K et al. Injury surveillance. *Injury Control and Safety Promotion*, 2003, 10:105–108.
7. Koornstra M et al. *Sunflower: a comparative study of the development of road safety in Sweden, the United Kingdom and the Netherlands*. Leidschendam, Institute for Road Safety Research, 2002.
8. Murray CJL, Lopez AD, eds. *The global burden of disease: a comprehensive assessment of mortality and disability from diseases, injuries, and risk factors in 1990 and projected to 2020*. Boston, MA, Harvard School of Public Health, 1996.
9. Bener A et al. Strategy to improve road safety in developing countries. *Saudi Medical Journal*, 2003, 24:447–452.
10. Nantulya VM, Reich MR. Equity dimensions of road traffic injuries in low- and middle-income countries. *Injury Control and Safety Promotion*, 2003, 10:13–20.
11. Vasconcellos E. Urban development and traffic accidents in Brazil. *Accident Analysis and Prevention*, 1999, 31:319–328.
12. Lamm R et al. Accidents in the U.S. and Europe. *Accident Analysis and Prevention*, 1985, 17:428–438.
13. *International Road Traffic Accident Database (IRTAD)* [online database]. Paris, Federal Highway Research Institute and the Organisation for Economic Co-operation and Development Road Transport Research Programme (http://www.bast.de/htdocs/fachthemen/irtad, accessed 7 November 2003).

14. Roberts I. Why have child pedestrian deaths fallen? *British Medical Journal*, 1993, 306:1737–1739.

15. Whitelegg J. *Transport for a sustainable future: the case for Europe*. London, Belhaven Press, 1993.

16. Tunali O. The billion-car accident waiting to happen. *World Watch*, 1996, 9:24–39.

17. Vasconcellos EA. Reassessing traffic accidents in developing countries. *Transport Policy*, 1996, 2:263–369.

18. *Mobility: prospects of sustainable mobility.* Geneva, World Council of Churches, 1998.

19. Breen J. Protecting pedestrians. *British Medical Journal*, 2002, 324:1109–1110.

20. Whitelegg J, Haq G. The global transport problem: same issues but a different place. In: Whitelegg J, Haq G, eds. *The Earthscan reader on world transport, policy and practice*. London, Earthscan Publications, 2003:1–28.

21. Smeed EW. Some statistical aspects of road safety research. *Journal of the Royal Statistical Society*, 1949, 1:1–23.

22. Jacobs GD, Hutchinson P. *A study of accident rates in developing countries*. Crowthorne, Transport and Road Research Laboratory, 1973 (TRRL Report LR 546).

23. Khayesi M. *An analysis of the pattern of road traffic accidents in relation to selected socio-economic dynamics and intervention measures in Kenya* [unpublished thesis]. Nairobi, Kenyatta University, 1999.

24. Bangdiwala SI et al. Statistical considerations for the interpretation of commonly utilized road traffic accident indicators: implications for developing countries. *Accident Analysis and Prevention*, 1985, 17:419–427.

25. Joksch HC. The relation between motor vehicle accident deaths and economic activity. *Accident Analysis and Prevention*, 1984, 16:207–210.

26. Wagenaar AC. Effects of macroeconomic conditions on the incidence of motor vehicle accidents. *Accident Analysis and Prevention*, 1984, 16:191–206.

27. Wintemute GJ. Is motor vehicle-related mortality a disease of development? *Accident Analysis and Prevention*, 1985, 17:223–237.

28. Partyka SC. Simple models of fatality trends using employment and population data. *Accident Analysis and Prevention*, 1984, 16:211–222.

29. Söderlund N, Zwi AB. Traffic-related mortality in industrialized and less developed countries. *Bulletin of the World Health Organization*, 1995, 73:175–182.

30. Odero W, Garner P, Zwi A. Road traffic injuries in developing countries: a comprehensive review of epidemiological studies. *Tropical Medicine and International Health*, 1997, 2:445–460.

31. Odero W, Khayesi M, Heda PM. Road traffic injuries in Kenya: magnitude, causes and status of intervention. *Injury Control and Safety Promotion*, 2003, 10:53–61.

32. Khayesi M. Liveable streets for pedestrians in Nairobi: the challenge of road traffic accidents. In: Whitelegg J, Haq G, eds. *The Earthscan reader on world transport, policy and practice*. London, Earthscan Publications, 2003:35–41.

33. Yang BM, Kim J. Road traffic accidents and policy interventions in Korea. *Injury Control and Safety Promotion*, 2003, 10:89–93.

34. Wang SY et al. Trends in road traffic crashes and associated injury and fatality in the People's Republic of China. *Injury Control and Safety Promotion*, 2003, 10:83–87.

35. Suriyanwongpaisal P, Kanchanasut S. Road traffic injuries in Thailand: trends, selected underlying determinants and status of intervention. *Injury Control and Safety Promotion*, 2003, 10:95–104.

36. Afukaar FK, Antwi P, Ofosu-Amah S. Pattern of road traffic injuries in Ghana: implications for control. *Injury Control and Safety Promotion*, 2003, 10:69–76.

37. Romao F et al. Road traffic injuries in Mozambique. *Injury Control and Safety Promotion*, 2003, 10:63–67.

38. Hijar M, Vasquez-Vela E, Arreola-Rissa C. Pedestrian traffic injuries in Mexico. *Injury Control and Safety Promotion*, 2003, 10:37–43.

39. Rodriguez DY, Fernandez FJ, Velasquez HA. Road traffic injuries in Colombia. *Injury Control and Safety Promotion*, 2003, 10:29–35.

40. St. Bernard G, Matthews W. A contemporary analysis of road traffic crashes, fatalities and injuries in Trinidad and Tobago. *Injury Control and Safety Promotion*, 2003, 10:21–27.

41. *Safety of vulnerable road users.* Paris, Organisation for Economic Co-operation and Development, 1998 (DSTI/DOT/RTR/RS7(98)1/FINAL) (http://www.oecd.org/dataoecd/24/4/2103492.pdf, accessed 17 November 2003).

42. Nantulya VM, Muli-Musiime F. Uncovering the social determinants of road traffic accidents in Kenya. In: Evans T et al., eds. *Challenging inequities: from ethics to action.* Oxford, Oxford University Press, 2001:211–225.

43. Nantulya VM, Reich MR. The neglected epidemic: road traffic injuries in developing countries. *British Medical Journal,* 2002, 324: 1139–1141.

44. Mohan D. Traffic safety and health in Indian cities. *Journal of Transport and Infrastructure,* 2002, 9: 79–94.

45. Barss P et al. *Injury prevention: an international perspective.* New York, NY, Oxford University Press, 1998.

46. Ryan GA, Ukai T. *Prevention and control of road traffic accidents: People's Republic of China* [assignment report]. Manila, World Health Organization Regional Office for the Western Pacific, 1988.

47. Sarin SM et al. Road accidents in India and other south east Asian countries [abstract]. *Journal of Traffic Medicine,* 1990, 18:316.

48. Lowe MD. *The bicycle: vehicle for a small planet.* Washington, DC, Worldwatch Institute, 1989 (Worldwatch Paper No. 90).

49. Li G, Baker SP. A comparison of injury death rates in China and the United States, 1986. *American Journal of Public Health,* 1991, 81:605–609.

50. Mohan D, Tiwari G. Road safety in low income countries: issues and concerns. In: *Reflections on the transfer of traffic safety knowledge to motorising nations.* Melbourne, Global Traffic Safety Trust, 1998:27–56.

51. *Traffic safety facts 2001: a compilation of motor vehicle crash data from the Fatality Analysis Reporting System and the General Estimates System.* Washington, DC, National Highway Traffic Safety Administration, National Center for Statistics and Analysis, 2002 (DOT HS-809-484).

52. *European social statistics: accidents at work and work-related health problems, 1994–2000.* Brussels, European Commission, 2002.

53. Murray W et al. *Evaluating and improving fleet safety in Australia.* Canberra, Australian Transport Safety Bureau, 2003.

54. Peden M, McGee K, Sharma G. *The injury chart book: a graphical overview of the global burden of injuries.* Geneva, World Health Organization, 2002.

55. Nantulya VM et al. Introduction: the global challenge of road traffic injuries: can we achieve equity in safety? *Injury Control and Safety Promotion,* 2003, 10:3–7.

56. *Cause of death.* Canberra, Australian Bureau of Statistics (various years).

57. Roberts I et al. Effect of environmental factors on risk of injury of child pedestrians by motor vehicles: a case-control study. *British Medical Journal,* 1995, 310:91–94.

58. Deal LW et al. Unintentional injuries in childhood: analysis and recommendations. *The Future of Children,* 2000, 10:4–22 (http://www.futureofchildren.org/usr_docvol10no1Art1.pdf, accessed 29 December 2003).

59. Fontaine H. Age des conducteurs de voiture et accidents de la route: quel risque pour les seniors? [Age of car drivers and road accidents: what is the risk for older people?] *Recherche, Transports, Sécurité,* 2003, 58:107–120.

60. Hakamies-Blomqvist L, Raitanen R, O'Neill D. Driver ageing does not cause higher accident rates per kilometre. *Transportation Research Part F: Traffic Psychology and Behaviour,* 2002, 5:271–274.

61. Mitchell K. Older persons and road safety: dispelling the myths. *World Transport Policy and Practice,* 2001, 8:17–26.

62. *Ageing and transport. Mobility needs and safety issues.* Paris, Organisation for Economic Co-operation and Development, 2001 (http://www1.oecd.org/publications/e-book/7701051E.pdf, accessed 17 November 2003).

63. *Annual health report 2002.* Qatar, Hamad Medical Corporation, 2002.

64. *Annual report 2000. Preventive medicine in 20 years, 1981–2000.* Abu Dhabi, United Arab Emirates Ministry of Health, Preventive Medicine Sector, 2003.

65. Peden MM. *Adult pedestrian traffic trauma in Cape Town with special reference to the role of alcohol* [unpublished thesis]. Cape Town, University of Cape Town, Department of Surgery, 1997.

66. Evans T, Brown H. Road traffic crashes: operationalizing equity in the context of health sector reform. *Injury Control and Safety Promotion*, 2003, 10:11–12.

67. LaFlamme L. *Social inequality in injury risks: knowledge accumulated and plans for the future.* Stockholm, National Institute of Public Health, 1998.

68. Roberts I, Power C. Does the decline in child injury death rates vary by social class? *British Medical Journal*, 1996, 313:784–786.

69. Hippisley-Cox J et al. Cross-sectional survey of socioeconomic variations in severity and mechanism of childhood injuries in Trent 1992–7. *British Medical Journal*, 2002, 324:1132–1134.

70. Whitlock G et al. Motor vehicle driver injury and marital status: a cohort study with prospective and retrospective injuries. *Journal of Epidemiology and Community Health*, 2003, 57:512–516.

71. Mohan D. Social cost of road traffic crashes in India. In: *Proceedings of the 1st Safe Community Conference on Cost of Injuries, Viborg, Denmark, 30 September – 3 October 2002.* Stockholm, Karolinska School of Public Health, 2003:33–38 (http://www.iitd.ernet.in/tripp/publications/paper/safety/dnmrk01.pdf, accessed 15 December 2003).

72. Thurman D. The epidemiology and economics of head trauma. In: Miller L, Hayes R, eds. *Head trauma: basic, preclinical, and clinical directions.* New York, NY, Wiley and Sons, 2001:327–347.

73. Baldo V et al. Epidemiological aspect of traumatic brain injury in Northeast Italy. *European Journal of Epidemiology*, 2003, 18:1059–1063.

74. Aare M, von Holst H. Injuries from motorcycle and moped crashes in Sweden from 1987 to 1999. *Injury Control and Safety Promotion*, 2003, 10:131–138.

75. Andrews CN, Kobusingye OC, Lett R. Road traffic accident injuries in Kampala. *East African Medical Journal*, 1999, 76:189–194.

76. Santikarn C, Santijiarakul S, Rujivipat V. The 2nd phase of the injury surveillance in Thailand. In: *Proceedings of the 4th International Conference on Measuring the Burden of Injury, Montreal, 16–17 May 2002.* Montreal, Canadian Association for Road Safety Professionals, 2002:77–86.

77. Solagberu B et al. Clinical spectrum of trauma at a university hospital in Nigeria. *European Journal of Trauma*, 2002, 6:365–369.

78. Blincoe L et al. *The economic impact of motor vehicle crashes, 2000.* Washington, DC, National Highway Traffic Safety Administration, 2002. (DOT HS-809-446)

79. Bakaitis SH. Economic consequences of traffic accidents in the Baltic countries. *Lituanus: Lithuanian Quarterly Journal of Arts and Sciences*, 2000, 46 (http://www.lituanus.org, accessed 17 November 2003).

80. Andersson A-L, Bunketorp O, Allebeck P. High rates of psychosocial complications after road traffic injuries. *Injury*, 1997, 28:539–543.

81. Fédération Européenne des Victimes de la Route [web site]. (http://www.fevr.org/english.html #Road, accessed 17 November 2003).

82. Mock CN et al. Economic consequences of injury and resulting family coping strategies in Ghana. *Accident Analysis and Prevention*, 2003, 35:81–90.

83. *Study of the physical, psychological and material secondary damage inflicted on the victims and their families by road crashes.* Geneva, Fédération Européenne des Victimes de la Route, 1993.

84. *Impact of road death and injury. Research into the principal causes of the decline in quality of life and living standard suffered by road crash victims and victim families. Proposals for improvements.* Geneva, Fédération Européenne des Victimes de la Route, 1997.

85. Mayou R, Bryant B, Duthie R. Psychiatric consequences of road traffic accidents. *British Medical Journal*, 1993, 307:647–651.

86. Mayou B, Bryant B. Outcome in consecutive emergency department attendees following a road traffic accident. *British Journal of Psychiatry*, 2001, 179:528–534.

87. Mayou R, Bryant B. Consequences of road traffic accidents for different types of road user. *Injury*, 2003, 34:197–202.

88. Dora C, Phillips M, eds. *Transport, environment and health.* Copenhagen, World Health Organization Regional Office for Europe, 2000 (European Series, No. 89) (http://www.who.dk/document/e72015.pdf, accessed 17 November 2003).

89. Wilkinson R, Marmot M, eds. *Social determinants of health: the solid facts,* 2nd ed. Copenhagen, World Health Organization Regional Office for Europe, 2003 (http://www.euro-who.int/document/e81384.pdf, accessed 17 November 2003).

90. *Transport accident costs and the value of safety.* Brussels, European Transport Safety Council, 1997.

91. *Transport safety performance in the EU: a statistical overview.* Brussels, European Transport Safety Council, 2003.

92. *Road crash costs in Australia.* Canberra, Bureau of Transport Economics, 2000 (Report 102).

93. Elvik R. How much do road accidents cost the national economy? *Accident Analysis and Prevention,* 2002, 32:849–851.

94. Babtie Ross Silcock, Transport Research Laboratory. *Guidelines for estimating the cost of road crashes in developing countries.* London, Department for International Development, 2003 (project R7780).

95. *The road to safety 2001–2005: building the foundations of a safe and secure road traffic environment in South Africa.* Pretoria, Ministry of Transport, 2001 (http://www.transport.gov.za/projects/index.html, accessed 17 November 2003).

96. Herbst AJ. The cost of medical and rehabilitation care for road accident victims at public hospitals. In: *Report of the Road Accident Fund Commission 2002.* Pretoria, Ministry of Transport, 2002:547–568 (http://www.transport.gov.za/library/docs/raf/annexJ.pdf, accessed 17 November 2003).

97. Benmaamar M. *Urban transport services in Sub-Saharan Africa: recommendations for reforms in Uganda.* Crowthorne, Transport Research Laboratory, 2002 (http://www.transportlinks.org/transport_links/filearea/publications/1_799_PA3834-02.pdf, accessed 7 November 2003).

98. Amonkou A et al. Economic incidence of road traumatology in Ivory Coast. *Urgences Médicales,* 1996, 15:197–200.

99. Zhou Y et al. Productivity loses from injury in China. *Injury Prevention,* 2003, 9:124–127.

100. Ad hoc Committee on Health Research Relating to Future Intervention Options. *Investing in health research and development.* Geneva, World Health Organization, 1996 (TDR/Gen/96.2).

101. Holder Y et al., eds. *Injury surveillance guidelines.* Geneva, World Health Organization, 2001 (WHO/NMH/VIP/01.02).

102. Sethi D et al., eds. *Guidelines for conducting community surveys on injuries and violence.* Geneva, World Health Organization, in press.

103. Blakstad F. Design of traffic accident recording systems. In: *United Nations Economic Commission for Africa: First African Road Safety Congress, Nairobi, Kenya, 27–30 August 1984.* Addis Ababa, United Nations Economic Commission for Africa, 1984:6.3–6.13.

104. *Model minimum uniform crash criteria. Final Report.* Washington, DC, Department of Transportation, 1998 (DOT HS-808-745).

105. Bartolomeos K, Peden M. The WHO-supported injury surveillance activities in Africa: Mozambique and Ethiopia. *African Safety Promotion Journal,* 2003, 1:34–37.

106. London J et al. Using mortuary statistics in the development of an injury surveillance system in Ghana. *Bulletin of the World Health Organization,* 2002, 80:357–364.

107. Ashley D, Holder Y. The Jamaican injury surveillance system: lessons learnt. *Injury Control and Safety Promotion,* 2002, 9:263–264.

108. Butchart A et al. The South African national non-natural mortality surveillance system: rationale, pilot results and evaluation. *South African Medical Journal,* 2001, 91:408–417.

109. Santikarn C et al. The establishment of injury surveillance in Thailand. *International Journal for Consumer and Product Safety,* 1999, 6:133–143.

110. Kobusingye OC, Lett RR. Hospital-based trauma registries in Uganda. *Journal of Trauma,* 2000, 48:498–502.

111. Chadbunchachai W et al. *Guidelines for post injury management, emergency medical service, and integrated trauma service.* Khon Kaen, Khon Kaen Regional Hospital, 1992.

112. Executive Committee for Health Development Planning. *The Health Development Plan in the Eighth National Economic and Social Development Plan (1997–2001).* Nonthaburi, Ministry of Public Health, 1997.

113. *Asia-Pacific Road Accident Database. User manual, version 1.1.* New York, NY, United Nations Economic

and Social Commission for Asia and the Pacific, 2002.

114. Ezenkwele UA, Holder Y. Applicability of CDC guidelines toward the development of an injury surveillance system in the Caribbean. *Injury Prevention*, 2001, 7:245–248.

115. *Community Road Accident Database (CARE)* [online database]. Brussels, European Commission, 2003 (http://europa.eu.int/comm/transport/care/, accessed 17 December 2003).

116. *Road safety guidelines for the Asian and Pacific region.* Manila, Asian Development Bank, 1997.

117. Mock CN et al. Incidence and outcome of injury in Ghana: a community-based survey. *Bulletin of the World Health Organization*, 1999, 77: 955–964.

118. Gururaj G. *Socio-economic impact of road traffic injuries. Collaborative study by National Institute of Mental Health and Neuro Science (NIMHANS), Transport Research Laboratory and Department for International Development.* Bangalore, National Institute of Mental Health and Neuro Science, 2001.

119. Ghaffar A. *National Injury Survey of Pakistan, 1997–1999.* Islamabad, National Injury Research Centre, 2001.

120. Butchart A, Kruger J, Lekoba R. Perceptions of injury causes and solutions in a Johannesburg township: implications for prevention. *Social Science and Medicine*, 2000, 50:331–344.

121. Kobusingye O, Guwatudde D, Lett R. Injury patterns in rural and urban Uganda. *Injury Prevention*, 2001, 7:46–50.

122. Hang HM et al. Community-based assessment of unintentional injuries: a pilot study in rural Vietnam. *Scandinavian Journal of Public Health*, 2003, 31:38–44.

123. *Fatality analysis reporting system (FARS): web-based encyclopedia*, Washington, DC, National Highway Traffic Safety Administration, 1996 (http://www-fars.nhtsa.dot.gov, accessed 17 December 2003).

124. Hardy BJ. *Analysis of pedestrian accidents, using police fatal accident files and SHIPS data.* Crowthorne, Transport Research Laboratory, 1997 (TRL Report No.282).

125. Baguley CJ. The importance of a road accident data system and its utilisation. In: *Proceedings of the International Symposium on Traffic Safety Strengthening and Accident Prevention, Nanjing, China, 28–30 November 2001.* Crowthorne, Transport Research Laboratory, 2001 (PA3807/02) (http://www.transport-links.org, accessed 27 November 2003).

126. *Statistical report of road accidents.* Kuala Lumpur, Royal Malaysia Police, 2001.

127. Hillman M et al. *One false move ... a study of children's independent mobility.* London, Policy Studies Institute, 1990.

128. Working Party on Passive Safety. *Preliminary report on the development of a global technical regulation concerning pedestrian safety.* Brussels, United Nations Economic Commission for Europe, Inland Transport Committee, 2003 (TRANS/WP.29/2003/99).

129. Mackay M. National differences in European mass accident data bases. In: *Proceedings of the Joint Session on Injury Scaling Issues, IRCOBI Annual Conference, Lisbon, September 2003,* in press.

130. Nakahara S, Wakai S. Underreporting of traffic injuries involving children in Japan. *Injury Prevention*, 2001, 7:242–244.

131. Leonard PA, Beattie TF, Gorman DR. Underrepresentation of morbidity from paediatric bicycle accidents by official statistics: a need for data collection in the accident and emergency department. *Injury Prevention*, 1999, 5: 303–304.

132. Gururaj G, Thomas AA, Reddi MN. Underreporting road traffic injuries in Bangalore: implications for road safety policies and programmes. In: *Proceedings of the 5th World Conference on Injury Prevention and Control.* New Delhi, Macmillan India, 2000:54 (Paper 1-3-I-04).

133. Mock CN, nii-Amon-Kotei D, Maier RV. Low utilization of formal medical services by injured persons in a developing nation: health service data underestimate the importance of trauma. *Journal of Trauma*, 1997, 42: 504–513.

134. Assum T. *Road safety in Africa: appraisal of road safety initiatives in five African countries.* Washington, DC, The World Bank and United Nations Economic Commission for Africa, 1998 (Working Paper No. 33).

135. *International statistical classification of diseases and related health problems,* tenth revision. *Volume 1: Tabular list; Volume 2: Instruction manual; Volume 3: Index.* Geneva, World Health Organization, 1994.

136. Joint Committee on Injury Scaling. *The Abbreviated Injury Scale: 1990 revision.* Chicago, IL, Association for the Advancement of Automotive Medicine, 1990.

CHAPTER 3

Risk factors

Introduction

In road traffic, risk is a function of four elements. The first is the exposure – the amount of movement or travel within the system by different users or a given population density. The second is the underlying probability of a crash, given a particular exposure. The third is the probability of injury, given a crash. The fourth element is the outcome of injury. This situation is summarized in Figure 3.1.

FIGURE 3.1

The main risk factors for road traffic injuries

Factors influencing exposure to risk
Economic factors, including social deprivation
Demographic factors
Land use planning practices which influence the length of a trip or travel mode choice
Mixture of high-speed motorized traffic with vulnerable road users
Insufficient attention to integration of road function with decisions about speed limits, road layout and design

Risk factors influencing crash involvement
Inappropriate or excessive speed
Presence of alcohol, medicinal or recreational drugs
Fatigue
Being a young male
Being a vulnerable road user in urban and residential areas
Travelling in darkness
Vehicle factors – such as braking, handling and maintenance
Defects in road design, layout and maintenance which can also lead to unsafe road user behaviour
Inadequate visibility due to environmental factors (making it hard to detect vehicles and other road users)
Poor road user eyesight

Risk factors influencing crash severity
Human tolerance factors
Inappropriate or excessive speed
Seat-belts and child restraints not used
Crash helmets not worn by users of two-wheeled vehicles
Roadside objects not crash protective
Insufficient vehicle crash protection for occupants and for those hit by vehicles
Presence of alcohol and other drugs

Risk factors influencing severity of post-crash injuries
Delay in detecting crash
Presence of fire resulting from collision
Leakage of hazardous materials
Presence of alcohol and other drugs
Difficulty rescuing and extracting people from vehicles
Difficulty evacuating people from buses and coaches involved in crash
Lack of appropriate pre-hospital care
Lack of appropriate care in the hospital emergency rooms

Risk arises largely as a result of various factors, that include (1):

— human error within the traffic system;
— the size and nature of the kinetic energy of the impact to which people in the system are exposed as a result of errors;
— the tolerance of the individual to this impact;
— the quality and availability of emergency services and acute trauma care.

The human operator often adapts to changing conditions in ways that do not always serve safety. A single error can have life or death consequences. Behind road-user errors, there are natural limitations. These include vision in night traffic, the detection of targets in the periphery of the eye, the estimation of speed and distance, the processing of information by the brain, and other physiological factors associated with age and sex that have a bearing on crash risk. Also influencing human error are external factors such as the design of the road, the design of the vehicle, traffic rules and the enforcement of traffic rules (2). Sophisticated and quality-assured systems that combine human beings and machines, therefore, need to have an in-built tolerance of human error (1).

The tolerance of the human body to the physical forces released in crashes is limited. Injury is broadly related to the kinetic energy applied to the human frame. The energy involved in a collision varies as the square of the velocity, so that small increases in speed result in major increases in the risk of injury. The relationship between impact forces in crashes and the injuries that are sustained is known for a number of parts of the body and type of injury – for different categories of road user, as well as for different age groups. Biomechanical thresholds associated with age, sex and speed are reliable predictors of crash injury. For example, impact forces that produce a moderate injury in a robust 25-year-old male will result in a life-threatening injury if applied to a 65-year-old infirm female (3).

The main road injury problems are being sustained worldwide by people who make similar mistakes, share the same human tolerance to injury limits and have the same inherent behavioural limitations. While the problems are different both qualitatively and quantitatively, the main risk factors appear to be the same worldwide (4,5).

Traditionally, analysis of risk has examined the road user, vehicle and road environment separately. In this report, a systems framework, where interactions between different components are taken into account, is used. Such a systems-oriented approach has been necessary for significant progress in tackling road trauma to be made (6).

Factors influencing exposure to risk

Risk in road traffic arises out of a need to travel – to have access to work, for instance, or for education or leisure pursuits. A range of factors determines who uses different parts of the transport system, how it is used and why, and at what times (7).

While in practical terms it may not be possible completely to eliminate all risk, it is possible to reduce the exposure to risk of severe injury and to minimize its intensity and consequences (1).

Rapid motorization
Motor vehicles

One of the main factors contributing to the increase in global road crash injury is the growing number of motor vehicles.

Since 1949, when Smeed (8) first demonstrated a relationship between fatality rates and motorization, several studies have shown a correlation between motor vehicle growth and the number of road crashes and injuries. While the motor vehicle and subsequent growth in the number of motor vehicles and road infrastructure has brought societal benefit, it has also led to societal cost to which road traffic injury contributes significantly. This explains why a number of studies are drawing attention to the need for careful consideration and planning of transport and mobility in view of the increasing motorization in different parts of the world (9–11).

Periods of economic prosperity tend to be associated with increasing mobility and demand for transport services. On the other hand, periods of economic decline lead to low generation of movement (12). In times of economic growth, traffic volumes increase, along with the number of crashes and injuries, and there are generally reductions in walking and cycling. Reductions in alcohol-related crashes have also been observed to coincide with periods of economic recession (13).

Motorization rate rises with income (14). In wealthier countries, there has been dramatic growth in the numbers of cars, but in many poorer countries the increases have been principally in motorcycles and minibuses. Some 80% of all cars are owned by 15% of the world's population, situated in North America, western Europe and Japan. Figure 3.2 and Table A.6 in the Statistical Annex both show that motorization is strongly correlated with income.

FIGURE 3.2

Motorization rate versus income[a]

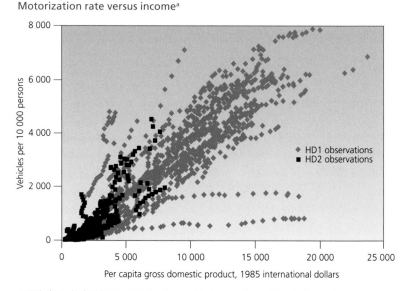

Per capita gross domestic product, 1985 international dollars

[a] HDI is the United Nations Human Development Index. Countries with an HDI more than 0.8 are labelled as HD1 while those with a value less than 0.8 are denoted as HD2.
Source: reproduced from reference 14, with minor editorial amendments, with the permission of the authors.

In China, where the economy is experiencing rapid growth, the number of vehicles has more than quadrupled since 1990, to over 55 million. In Thailand, between 1987 and 1997, there was an almost four-fold increase in the number of registered motor vehicles, from 4.9 million to 17.7 million (*15*). In India, the number of four-wheeled motor vehicles increased by 23% to 4.5 million between 1990 and 1993. All of these figures are far below the rates of car ownership per capita in high-income countries (*16*). It is predicted that the motor vehicle numbers for countries of the Organisation for Economic Co-operation and Development (OECD) could increase up to 62% by the year 2015, to a total of 705 million (*14*).

Motor vehicle growth in low-income countries is taking place against a background of associated problems. Only a small number of people in these countries can afford cars, while the costs of roads, parking spaces, air pollution and road traffic injuries are borne by the whole society (*9*). Despite the rapid growth in motorized traffic, most families in low-income and middle-income countries are unlikely to own a car within the next 25 years (*5*). In terms of exposure to risk, the main modes of travel in these countries in the foreseeable future are likely to remain walking, cycling and public transport. This emphasizes the importance of planning for the needs of these road users, who, as was seen in Chapter 2, bear a high proportion of the burden of road traffic injuries.

The case of reunification in Germany provides a good illustration of how economic factors can influence crash injury. Here, overnight, many people suddenly experienced a surge in affluence and access to previously unavailable cars. In the two years following reunification, the number of cars that were bought and the total distance travelled by cars increased by over 40%. At the same time, between 1989 and 1991, there was a four-fold increase in death rates for car occupants, with an eleven-fold increase for those aged 18–20 years. The overall death rate in road crashes in this period nearly doubled, from 4 per 100 000 population in 1989 to 8 per 100 000 in 1991 (*17*). Other countries where motor vehicle growth has been shown to be associated with an increase in road traffic injuries are the Czech Republic, Hungary and Poland (*11, 18*). In Poland, for every additional 1000 cars purchased between 1989 and 1991, an additional 1.8 traffic fatalities and 27 people injured in crashes were recorded (*11*).

Traffic volume is a particularly important risk factor for injuries among child pedestrians. Roberts et al. have shown that when traffic volumes fall there is a reduction in child pedestrian death rates (*19, 20*).

Buses and trucks are a major mode of travel in low-income and middle-income countries. High volumes of passengers being transported have an impact on the safety, not only of the passengers themselves, but also on vulnerable road users. In New Delhi, buses and trucks are involved in almost two thirds of crashes involving vulnerable road users, and these people make up over 75% of all road traffic deaths (*5*).

Motorized two-wheeled vehicles

Although the greatest growth rate in the number of motor vehicles is expected in Asian countries, most of the increase in vehicle fleets is likely to be in motorized two-wheeled vehicles and three-wheelers (*5*). In many such places, it is estimated that motorized two-wheelers will comprise between 40% and 70% of the total vehicle fleet.

In south-east Asia, there are several countries with a large proportion of two-wheeled and three-wheeled vehicles whose growth in numbers has been associated with a large rise in road traffic injuries. Examples are Cambodia (where 75% of all vehicles are motorized two-wheelers or motorized three-wheelers), the Lao People's Democratic Republic (79%), Malaysia (51%) and Viet Nam (95%). In Viet Nam, the number of motorcycles grew by 29% during 2001; at the same time road deaths rose by 37% (*21*). An increase in use of motorized two-wheelers in China, Province of Taiwan, where such vehicles comprise 65% of all registered motor vehicles, was also associated with increasing deaths and injuries (*22*).

In the United Kingdom, after a long-term downward trend in both motorized two-wheeler traffic and deaths related to their use, a resurgence of interest in these vehicles over the last few years has been accompanied by sharp increases in motorized two-wheeler deaths and serious injuries. The national level of deaths and serious injuries among users of motorized two-wheelers in 2001 was 21% above the average for 1994–1998 (23).

Like other motor vehicles, motorized two-wheelers also cause injuries to other road users. In low-income countries, where the majority of pedestrian impacts are with buses and cars, one hospital-based study in New Delhi found that 16% of injured pedestrians had been struck by motorized two-wheelers (24).

Non-motorized traffic

Non-motorized vehicles predominate in both rural and urban areas in some low-income and middle-income countries. In these countries, the proportion of road traffic injuries from non-motorized forms of travel varies according to the way motorized and non-motorized modes of travel are split (11). In Asia, however, motorcycles are dominant, which partly explains the high proportion of motorcycle fatalities and injuries. Generally speaking in developing countries, pedestrian and cyclist traffic has grown without accompanying improvements in facilities for these road users. The high number of pedestrian and cyclist casualties in these countries reflects not only their inherent vulnerability but also insufficient attention to their needs in policy-making (11, 25, 26).

Demographic factors

Different groups of people have different exposures to risk. As populations change over time, so the overall exposure of that population will change. Fluctuations in the relative sizes of different population groups will have a strong effect on the road traffic toll. For instance, in industrialized countries, young drivers and riders – at increased risk of involvement in road crashes – are currently overrepresented in casualty figures. Demographic changes, though, in these countries over the next 20–30 years will result in road users over 65 years of age becoming the largest group of road users. Their physical vulnerability, though, places them at high risk of fatal and serious injuries (27). In low-income countries, the expected demographic evolution suggests that younger road users will continue to be the predominant group involved in road crashes.

In some high-income countries, more than 20% of the population will be 65 years or above by 2030 (28). Despite the rising number of older people holding driving licences in such countries, their declining driving ability as well as possible financial constraints will mean that many of them will have to give up driving. In many low-income countries, older people may never have driven in the first place. Worldwide, a large proportion of older people will still be dependent on public transport or will walk. This illustrates the importance of providing safer and shorter pedestrian routes and safe and convenient public transport.

Transport, land use and road network planning

Planning decisions regarding transport, land use and road networks have significant effects on public health – as they affect the amount of air pollution by vehicles, the degree of physical exercise undertaken by individuals, and the volume of road traffic crashes and injuries.

The development of a network of roads – or indeed of other forms of transport, such as railways – has a profound effect on communities and individuals. It influences such things as economic activity, property prices, air and noise pollution, social deprivation and crime – in addition to health. Long commuting times degrade the quality of life and therefore health. Sedentary travel directly and adversely affects health (29).

In the absence of proper land-use planning, residential, commercial and industrial activity will evolve in a haphazard pattern, and road traffic will evolve similarly to meet the needs of these various activities. This is likely to produce heavy flows of traffic through residential areas, vehicles capable of high speed mixing with pedestrians, and heavy, long-distance commercial traffic using routes not designed for such vehicles. The consequent exposure to traffic injury can be high for car occupants, and even more so for vulnerable road users, such as pedestrians, cyclists and motorized two-wheeler users (*30*).

The mixed nature of road traffic in many low-income and middle-income countries – with pedestrians, bicycles, handcarts, mopeds, motorcycles, vans, cars, trucks and buses in different proportions – means that many of the technical aspects of planning, highway design, traffic engineering and traffic management need to be worked out locally, rather than being imported. For example, in many Asian cities, with some notable exceptions, the road network is used by at least seven categories of motorized and non-motorized vehicles, of varying widths and speeds, all sharing the road space. There is generally no effective channelling or segregation of the different categories, or speed control (*31*).

Where planning of land use does take place, it is often done with a view to creating efficient flows of traffic, resulting in major arterial, high-speed routes that cut off different urban sections, to the disadvantage of local residents. Environmental criteria – such as reductions in noise, pollution and visual intrusion – are also often employed in planning. Safety considerations are brought in much less often. When safety criteria are applied to land use planning, though, there is ample evidence of significant reductions in exposure to traffic injury (*29*).

Increased need for travel

All growing urban areas experience a movement of residents from the inner districts to the suburbs. Socioeconomic changes in many places are leading to a profusion of out-of-town supermarkets and shopping malls, with a consequent loss of local shops. Both of these phenomena generate increased traffic, less opportunity for travel by public transport, and increased exposure to risk.

These factors need to be better recognized and evaluated in planning processes. This applies not only to developed countries but also to developing countries, some of which contain rapidly-growing megacities, with their significant but undocumented changes in patterns of wealth and living space.

Choice of less safe forms of travel

Of the four main modes of travel, road travel scores by far the highest risk in most countries – using almost any measure of exposure – compared with rail, air and marine travel (*32, 33*).

Within the mode of road travel, major variations in risk exist between pedestrians, cyclists, riders of motorized two-wheelers, car occupants, and bus and truck passengers. The risks for these road users also vary greatly according to the traffic mix and hence vary greatly from country to country. In general, in high-income countries, riders of motorized two-wheelers have the highest levels of risk.

In European Union countries, the risk of death for motorized two-wheeler users is 20 times that of car occupants (see Table 3.1). Travelling by car is some 7–9 times safer than cycling or walking, but car occupants are still 10 times less safe than bus occupants. All these relative risks are calculated on the basis of distance travelled. Even when the risks of walking or cycling before or after a train or bus trip are taken into account, travel by public transport is still safer than car travel, when the collective safety of all users is considered (*32*).

TABLE 3.1

Deaths per 100 million passenger-kilometres versus passenger-travel hours in European Union countries for the period 2001–2002

	Deaths per 100 million passenger-kilometres[a]	Deaths per 100 million passenger-travel hours[b]
Roads (total)	0.95	28
Powered two-wheelers	13.8	440
Foot	6.4	75
Cycle	5.4	25
Car	0.7	25
Bus and coach	0.07	2
Ferry	0.25	16
Air (civil aviation)	0.035	8
Rail	0.035	2

[a] Passenger-kilometres is the total distance covered by all the individuals travelling on that mode.

[b] Passenger-travel hours is the total time spent by all the individuals travelling on that mode.

Source: reproduced from reference *32*, with minor editorial amendments, with the permission of the publisher.

The choice of mode of travel is greatly influenced by the climate. Extremes of temperature severely limit cycling and walking.

As Table 3.2 shows, the traffic crash cost of injuries among motorized two-wheeler users is also higher than for any other mode (*33*).

TABLE 3.2

Traffic crash cost per passenger-kilometres

Mode of transport	Cost per passenger- km (in US$)
Commercial aviation	0.01
Rail	0.06
Bus	0.23
Car	0.28
General aviation	0.39
Motorcycle	1.52

Source: reproduced from reference *33,* with the permission of the publisher.

The level and mix of motorized two-wheeler use have long been volatile features of road use, both for urban commuting and for rural recreation (*34*). In this context, if the number of road injuries is to be minimized, care should be taken to avoid the adoption of policies which could encourage the growth of motorized two-wheeler traffic by giving advantages to motorized two-wheeler users.

A recent report by the organization Transport for London stated that one reason for providing motorized two-wheelers with exemption from the city's congestion charge scheme was their smaller contribution to congestion in central London. Transport for London suggested that there could be a small increase in motorized two-wheeler activity as a consequence of the new scheme, though it stated that distinguishing such a change from background trends could be difficult (*35*). When compared against trends over recent years for all other vehicle types, though, the relative share of trips undertaken by motorized two-wheelers was already increasing (*35*), and motorized two-wheeler users are a leading casualty group in the United Kingdom. By the end of 2002, deaths and serious injuries among motorized two-wheeler users in London were 31% above the 1994–1998 average (*36*). Thus if present trends continue, it seems unlikely that the target of a 40% reduction in motorcycle deaths by 2010 will be achieved.

Risk factors influencing crash involvement
Speed

The speed of motor vehicles is at the core of the road injury problem. Speed influences both crash risk and crash consequence.

"Excess speed" is defined as a vehicle exceeding the relevant speed limit; "inappropriate speed" refers to a vehicle travelling at a speed unsuitable for the prevailing road and traffic conditions. While speed limits only declare higher speeds to be illegal it remains for each driver and rider to decide the appropriate speed within the limit.

The speed drivers choose to travel at is influenced by many factors (see Table 3.3). Modern cars have high rates of acceleration and can easily reach very high speeds in short distances. The physical layout of the road and its surroundings can both encourage and discourage speed. Crash risk increases as speed increases, especially at road junctions and while overtaking – as road users underestimate the speed, and overestimate the distance, of an approaching vehicle.

TABLE 3.3

Examples of factors affecting drivers' choice of speed

Road and vehicle related	Traffic and environment related	Driver related
Road	Traffic	Age
Width	Density	Sex
Gradient	Composition	Reaction time
Alignment	Prevailing speed	Attitudes
Surroundings	Environment	Thrill-seeking
Layout	Weather	Risk acceptance
Markings	Surface condition	Hazard perception
Surface quality	Natural light	Alcohol level
Vehicle	Road lighting	Ownership of vehicle
Type	Signs	Circumstances of
Power/weight ratio	Speed limit	journey
Maximum speed	Enforcement	Occupancy of vehicle
Comfort		

Source: reproduced from reference *37,* with the permission of the publisher.

Crash risk

There is a large amount of evidence of a significant relationship between mean speed and crash risk:

- The probability of a crash involving an injury is proportional to the square of the speed. The probability of a serious crash is proportional to the cube of the speed. The probability of a fatal crash is related to the fourth power of the speed (38, 39).
- Empirical evidence from speed studies in various countries has shown that an increase of 1 km/h in mean traffic speed typically results in a 3% increase in the incidence of injury crashes (or an increase of 4–5% for fatal crashes), and a decrease of 1 km/h in mean traffic speed will result in a 3% decrease in the incidence of injury crashes (or a decrease of 4–5% for fatal crashes) (40).
- Taylor et al. (41, 42), in their study on different types of roads in the United Kingdom, concluded that for every 1 mile/h (1.6 km/h) reduction in average traffic speed, the highest reduction achievable in the volume of crashes was 6% (in the case of urban roads with low average speeds). These are typically busy main roads in towns with high levels of pedestrian activity, wide variations in speeds and high frequencies of crashes.
- A meta-analysis of 36 studies on speed limit changes showed, at levels above 50 km/h, a decrease of 2% in the number of crashes for every 1 km/h reduction in the average speed (43).
- A variation in speeds between different vehicles travelling at different speeds within the traffic stream is also associated with crash occurrence (44).
- A study of crashes within rural 60 km/h zones involving injuries to car occupants found that the relative risk of crash involvement doubles, or more, for each increase of 5 km/h of travelling speed above 60 km/h (45) (see Table 3.4). Travelling at 5 km/h above a road speed limit of 60 km/h results in an increase in the relative risk of being involved in a casualty crash that is comparable with having a blood alcohol concentration (BAC) of 0.05 gram per decilitre (g/dl) (45).

TABLE 3.4

Relative risks of involvement in a casualty crash for speed and alcohol

Speed (km/h)	Speed (relative risk[a])	Blood alcohol concentration (g/dl)	Blood alcohol concentration (relative risk[b])
60	1.0	0.00	1.0
65	2.0	0.05	1.8
70	4.2	0.08	3.2
75	10.6	0.12	7.1
80	31.8	0.21	30.4

[a] Relative to a sober driver travelling at the speed limit of 60 km/h.
[b] Relative to driving with a zero blood alcohol concentration.
Source: reproduced from reference 45 with the permission of the publisher.

Severity of crash injuries

Speed has an exponentially detrimental effect on safety. As speeds increase, so do the number and severity of injuries. Studies show that the higher the impact speed, the greater the likelihood of serious and fatal injury:

- For car occupants, the severity of crash injury depends on the change of speed during the impact, usually denoted as Δv. As Δv increases from about 20 km/h to 100 km/h, the probability of fatal injuries increases from close to zero to almost 100% (46).
- The probability of serious injury for belted front-seat occupants is three times as great at 30 miles/h (48 km/h) and four times as great at 40 miles/h (64 km/h), compared with the risk at 20 miles/h (32 km/h) (47).
- For car occupants in a crash with an impact speed of 50 miles/h (80 km/h), the likelihood of death is 20 times what it would have been at an impact speed of 20 miles/h (32 km/h) (48).
- Pedestrians have a 90% chance of surviving car crashes at 30 km/h or below, but less than a 50% chance of surviving impacts at 45 km/h or above (49, 50) (see Figure 3.3).
- The probability of a pedestrian being killed rises by a factor of eight as the impact speed of the car increases from 30 km/h to 50 km/h (51).
- Older pedestrians are even more physically vulnerable as speeds increase (52) (see Figure 3.4).
- Excess and inappropriate speed contributes to around 30% of fatal crashes in high-income countries (53).

FIGURE 3.3

Pedestrian fatality risk as a function of the impact speed of a car

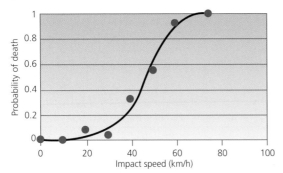

Source: reproduced from reference *49*, with the permission of the publisher.

FIGURE 3.4

Fatal injury rates by vehicle speed and pedestrian age in Florida, 1993–1996 (pedestrians in single-vehicle crashes)

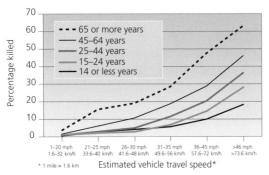

Source: reproduced from reference *52*, with minor editorial amendments, with the permission of the publisher.

In China, in 1999, speed was the main reported cause of road traffic crashes (*54*). Errors – such as loss of control of vehicle, speeding, misjudgement and improper overtaking – contributed to 44% of all police-reported crashes in Kenya (*55*). Speed was identified as the main contributory factor in 50% of road crashes in Ghana between 1998 and 2000 (*56*).

Speed has also been identified as an important factor in crashes involving commercial road transport and public passenger vehicles (*55, 57*). In South Africa, for instance, 50% of such crashes are related to speed (*57*). While in many high-income countries, there is increasing use of in-built mechanisms

in trucks and buses to restrict speeds above a certain limit, such devices are frequently resisted in low-income and middle-income countries for commercial reasons, or else, if installed, are disabled by the operators. Commercial operations are often based on timetables that put pressure on drivers to speed. In many low-income and middle-income countries, the pay of bus drivers is related to ticket receipts, which encourages high speeds (*58*).

Everywhere, speed limits are widely flouted (*37*). At high speeds, environmental damage from exhaust emissions and traffic noise are greater at higher than at moderate speeds.

Figure 3.5 summarizes the main effects of speed on the risk of crashes and crash injury.

FIGURE 3.5

Summary of the effects of speed on crashes and crash injury

In highly-motorized countries, excessive and inappropriate speed is a major cause of around one in three of all fatal and serious crashes (*53*). Speed affects the risk of a crash occurring: the greater the speed, the less time there is to prevent a collision. At the same time, the greater the speed, the more severe the consequences, once a crash has occurred. Various studies have indicated that:

■ An average increase in speed of 1 km/h is associated with a 3% higher risk of a crash involving an injury (*40, 41*).

■ In severe crashes, the increased risk is even greater. In such cases, an average increase in speed of 1 km/h leads to a 5% higher risk of serious or fatal injury (*40, 41*).

■ Travelling at 5 km/h above a road speed limit of 65 km/h results in an increase in the relative risk of being involved in a casualty crash that is comparable with having a BAC of 0.05 g/dl (*45*).

■ For car occupants in a crash with an impact speed of 50 miles/h (80 km/h), the likelihood of death is 20 times what it would have been at an impact speed of 20 miles/h (32 km/h) (*48*).

■ Pedestrians have a 90% chance of surviving car crashes at 30km/h or below, but less than a 50% chance of surviving impacts at 45 km/h or above (*50*).

■ The probability of a pedestrian being killed rises by a factor of 8 as the impact speed of the car increases from 30 km/h to 50 km/h (*51*).

Pedestrians and cyclists

A disproportionately large number of pedestrian

crashes and cyclist crashes occur in low-income countries (4, 59–61). Pedestrian casualties also represent a huge cost to society in industrialized nations (62), where the risks (measured in distance travelled or time spent travelling) are many more times higher for pedestrians and cyclists than for car users (63).

The crash risks incurred by pedestrians and cyclists result from a complex mix of factors. A fundamental factor in high-income countries is the fact that the modern traffic system is designed largely from the perspective of a motor vehicle user (64). Provision for pedestrians and cyclists in low-income countries is rudimentary or even non-existent.

The principal risk factor for unprotected road users is the mixing of unprotected people with motor vehicles capable of high speeds (5, 60, 65). The survival of unprotected users depends upon ensuring either that they are separated from the high speeds of motor vehicles or – in the more common situation of shared use of the road – that the vehicle speed at the point of collision is low enough to prevent serious injury on impact with crash-protective safer car fronts. The absence of adequate separate pedestrian and cyclist facilities, such as footpaths or cycle tracks, creates a high risk for these road users.

If separation is not possible, road management and vehicle speed management are essential. At low speeds, drivers have more time to react to unexpected events and to avoid collisions. At speeds of less than 30 km/h, pedestrians and cyclists can mix with motor vehicles in relative safety (51). Poor provision at crossings and junctions is also a feature of unsafe shared use. In urban areas, most fatal or serious cyclist crashes occur at junctions (66).

Other risk factors for pedestrians and cyclists include:
— poor street visibility;
— poor understanding on the part of pedestrians of road safety; in a study in Jordan, nearly half of children crossing a road did not check for oncoming traffic even once before or while crossing (67);

— alcohol impairment on the part of the cyclists or pedestrians;
— poor design of the fronts of cars (65, 68–71).

Young drivers and riders

Globally, road crash injury is a leading cause of death for young drivers and riders (72). Both young age and inexperience contribute to the high risk of these drivers and riders. Young drivers have a higher crash risk than older drivers (73). Being a young male is also predictive of crash involvement as a driver. It has been established in industrialized countries that men, especially young men in their first few years of driving, have higher rates of crash involvement than women, even when corrected for exposure factors (74).

In a study of injuries in Australia, Japan, Malaysia and Singapore, the highest injury risk was found among motorcyclists with a provisional licence, followed by those in their first year of riding (75).

The crash risks for teenage drivers are greater than those for any other comparable age group, with 16-year-old and 17-year-old drivers being at particular risk (76). Studies in developed countries indicate that the risks were particularly high during the 12 months after a full licence had been issued (76). The factors behind the elevated risk include:
— mobility patterns and vehicle characteristics (e.g. the vehicle is often borrowed);
— psychological characteristics, such as thrill-seeking and over-confidence;
— less tolerance of alcohol compared with older people;
— excess or inappropriate speed, the most common error among young drivers and riders.

Late-night driving is also a predictive factor for serious crashes among young drivers. For 16-year-old drivers, the late-night risk is three times the daytime risk (see also Box 3.1). While the night-time risks are greater for the youngest drivers, it is among drivers aged 20–44 years that the ratio of night-time driving risk to daytime risk is greatest – by a factor of four (76).

BOX 3.1

The human consequences of speed

Joelle Sleiman is 21 years old and lives in Marjeyoun in southern Lebanon. Her family – including her parents and two younger brothers – managed to survive the long civil war without serious incidents. On 16 August 2001, though, they were struck by tragedy when the two sons – Nicolas, 17 years, and Andy, 16 years – were involved in a car crash.

Nicolas loved cars and fast driving. Because of the lack of law enforcement in their area he was able to take the car out without a licence and drive at high speeds. He didn't listen to his parents' pleas not to drive.

On that terrible night, Joelle's mother was watching television late, waiting for the boys to come home. Instead, news of the crash arrived. Joelle and her parents rushed to the hospital, where they found Andy dead and Nicolas in a grave condition, not responding to treatment. They managed, with difficulty, to have Nicolas transferred to a hospital in Beirut, where he lay in a coma.

On the same day that Andy's funeral was held, the father was told that Nicolas's prospects were not promising. The family spent the next week praying for a miracle, but nothing could be done. Nicolas died one week after his brother. It eventually emerged that the boys were trying to avoid an unknown driver coming at them in the wrong direction, when they hit a wall.

When Joelle talks to other teenagers about speeding, they sometimes say to her, "It is up to us if we choose to die". They forget, Joelle points out, that they are not the only ones affected, that there are parents, brothers, sisters and close friends who love them. They should also think about that.

Losing her two brothers has completely changed Joelle's life. She now lives alone at home with her parents. She joined the Youth Association for Social Awareness (YASA), which has helped ease her inner pain. While she will not get her brothers back, she says that at least she can help other sisters avoid what she went through. Her work with YASA gives her pride, and she does it thinking of Andy and Nicolas.

The risk for young drivers increases exponentially as the number of passengers increases (76). One case–control study indicated that a third of all crashes involving young drivers might have been prevented if young drivers had been restricted to driving with no more than one passenger (77).

Alcohol

Crash risk

A case–control study carried out in Michigan, United States, in 1964, known as the Grand Rapids study (78), showed that drivers who had consumed alcohol had a higher risk of involvement in crashes than those with a zero BAC and that this risk increased rapidly with BAC. These results provided the basis for the future setting of legal blood alcohol limits and breath content limits in many countries around the world, typically at 0.08 g/dl.

In 1981, an Australian study found that the risk of crash involvement was 1.83 times greater at a BAC of 0.05 g/dl than at a BAC of zero (79). Re-analysis of the Grand Rapids data by Hurst et al. (80) also concluded that the risks associated with lower BAC levels were greater than originally thought. This information, together with findings from behavioural and experimental studies (81), provided a justification for many countries to reduce their legal BAC limits to 0.05 g/dl.

A major case–control study – using more robust research design and multivariate analytical techniques than the Grand Rapids study – has recently taken place to determine at what level of BAC an elevated crash risk begins (82). This study, involving 14 985 drivers, was conducted in the United States at Long Beach, California and Fort Lauderdale, Florida. The overall result was in agreement with previous studies showing increasing relative risk as levels of BAC increased (see Figure 3.6). The study found that the relative risk of crash involvement starts to increase significantly at a BAC level of 0.04 g/dl.

FIGURE 3.6

Relative risk of driver involvement in police-reported crashes

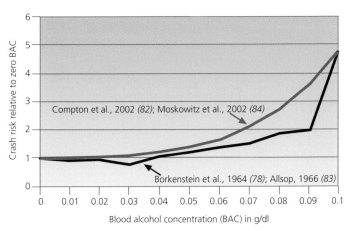

Source: references 78, 82–84.

An Australian study of alcohol and motorcycle crashes found that having a BAC level greater than zero was associated with five times the risk relative to a zero BAC (85).

Age of drivers

The risk of a crash with alcohol varies with age and drinking experience. Zador estimated that crash rates of male drivers aged 16–20 years were at least three times the estimated crash rate of male drivers aged 25 years and above, for every BAC level (86). With few exceptions, the relative risk of being fatally injured in a single-vehicle crash was found to decrease with increasing driver age for every BAC level, for both men and women (87).

A study on drivers killed in road crashes estimated that teenage drivers had more than five times the risk of a crash compared with drivers aged 30 and above, at all levels of BAC. Drivers in the 20–29 years age group were estimated to have a three times higher risk than drivers aged 30 years and above, at all BAC levels (88). Teenage drivers with a BAC of 0.03 g/dl carrying two or more passengers were 34 times more at risk of a crash than drivers aged 30 years or more, with zero BAC, driving with one passenger (88).

Severity of crashes

A study in the United States of relative fatality risks at different BAC levels indicated that for single-vehicle crashes, each 0.02% increase in BAC level approximately doubled the risk of involvement in a fatal crash (86). A similar finding was reported in a New Zealand study that used a sample of crashes involving mainly single vehicles. The study calculated the risk for a driver of a fatal injury during the night-time, according to the number of passengers in the vehicle, the driver's age and the driver's BAC level (88).

A study in the United Kingdom, comparing data from roadside surveys with the corresponding ranges of BAC levels collected from coroners' reports, showed that the relative fatality risk increases exponentially with BAC, and that this risk was an order of magnitude larger than the risk of being involved in a crash with injuries (89).

The frequency of drinking and driving varies considerably around the world. Despite that, and despite the fact that there have been few studies in low-income countries, research indicates that the phenomenon continues to be a major risk factor in traffic crashes. After many years of decline, the rate of road traffic deaths involving alcohol has begun rising in several high-income countries (90). A review of surveys of drinking and driving levels in traffic in European Union countries found that alcohol was present in between 1% and 3% of drivers (91). Roadside surveys taken in Croatia indicated that over 4% of drivers were intoxicated (92). A Ghanaian study found that over 7% of drivers in a random breath test had BAC levels above 0.08 g/dl (93). In New Delhi, India, a study showed that a third of motorized two-wheeler riders taken to hospital admitted to driving under the influence of alcohol (94).

The effects of alcohol consumption on the risk of crashes and of crash injury are summarized in Figure 3.7.

FIGURE 3.7

Effects of alcohol on risk of crashes and on crash injury

- Drivers and motorcyclists with any level of BAC greater than zero are at higher risk of a crash than those whose BAC is zero.

- For the general driving population, as the BAC increases from zero, the risk of being involved in a crash starts to rise significantly at a BAC of 0.04 g/dl (82).

- Inexperienced young adults driving with a BAC of 0.05 g/dl have 2.5 times the risk of a crash compared with more experienced drivers (95).

- A study on drivers killed in road crashes estimated that teenage drivers had more than five times the risk of a crash compared with drivers aged 30 and above, at all levels of BAC. Drivers 20–29 years old were estimated to have three times the risk compared with drivers aged 30 years and above, at all BAC levels (88).

- Teenage drivers with a BAC of 0.03 g/dl carrying two or more passengers were 34 times more at risk of a crash than drivers aged 30 years or more, with zero BAC, driving with one passenger (88).

- If a BAC limit is fixed at 0.10 g/dl, this will result in three times the risk of a crash that exists with the most common limit, in high-income countries, of 0.05 g/dl. If the legal limit stands at 0.08 g/dl, there will still be twice the risk that there would be with a limit of 0.05 g/dl.

- Alcohol consumption by drivers puts pedestrians and riders of motorized two-wheelers at risk.

Research on the role of alcohol in crashes

Apart from in those countries where alcohol is prohibited, impairment by alcohol is likely to be an important factor in causing crashes and in exacerbating the consequences of crashes. Systematic surveillance, though, is not established in many countries (96, 97). In many low-income countries, the police often lack the means, in terms of human resources and equipment, to monitor routinely the level of alcohol in drivers, even where legal limits exist (96).

As Odero and Zwi (97) for low-income and middle-income countries and the European Transport Safety Council (ETSC) for Europe (91) have outlined, variable measurements; testing for different injury severities and different thresholds for BAC (where they exist), preclude a full comparison of excess alcohol levels between countries. Some studies refer to presence of any alcohol, others to alcohol over the legal limit, where such a limit exists.

From an investigation of studies conducted in low-income countries, it emerged that alcohol was present in between 33% and 69% of fatally-injured drivers, and in between 8% and 29% of drivers involved in crashes who were not fatally injured (97). Peden et al. (98) found that alcohol was a factor in around 29% of non-fatally-injured drivers, and in over 47% of fatally-injured drivers in South Africa. A later study found excess alcohol in over 52% of trauma patients involved in road crashes (99) (see also Box 3.2).

BOX 3.2

Alcohol-related road traffic deaths in South Africa

According to the South African national injury mortality surveillance system, there were 25 361 fatal injuries registered at 32 state mortuaries in 2001. This represents approximately 35% of all non-natural mortality in South Africa in that year. Transport-related deaths accounted for 27% of all the fatal injuries. Pedestrians were the group of road users most frequently killed (37.3%), followed by passengers of vehicles (17.4%), drivers (14.0%) and cyclists (3.1%).

Alcohol is a major risk factor for all types of fatal road traffic injury in South Africa. Tests for BAC were conducted on 2372 (or 34.6%) of the 6859 transport-related deaths. More than half (51.9%) of all transport-related deaths had elevated BAC, and of these positive cases, 91% recorded BAC levels of 0.05 g/dl or higher.

Pedestrians, followed by drivers, were most likely to be BAC-positive (see table below).

BOX 3.2 (continued)

	Blood alcohol concentration (g/dl)				
	Zero (%)	0.01–0.04 (%)	0.05–0.14 (%)	0.15–0.24 (%)	≥0.25 (%)
Pedestrians	37.5	5.4	12.0	20.5	24.7
Passengers	62.6	4.7	14.0	13.7	5.0
Drivers	48.2	5.3	18.2	18.8	9.5
Cyclists	61.3	3.2	15.1	14.0	6.5

Pedestrian fatalities also had the highest mean BAC levels (0.20 g/dl). Over 50% of drivers killed had elevated BAC levels and the mean level for drivers – 0.17 g/dl – was over three times the legal limit for driving, currently set in South Africa at 0.05 g/dl.

Research in the United States indicates that motorized two-wheeler riders have higher intoxication rates than motor vehicle drivers (*100*).

In Sweden, the Netherlands and the United Kingdom, the proportion of fatally-injured drivers with excess alcohol for each country is around 20%, though the legal limits in these countries differ considerably, being 0.02 g/dl, 0.05 g/dl and 0.08 g/dl, respectively (*101*).

Perception of risk of being caught with excess alcohol

Research has shown that the only consistently effective strategy for dealing with the problem of excess alcohol is to increase the perceived risk of being caught. Such a perception is considered a better deterrent than the severity or the swiftness of the penalty (*102*). With a few exceptions – including Australia and the Nordic countries – both the perception and the actual likelihood of being detected for excess alcohol are low in most countries, irrespective of personal income (*91*). In Thailand, over 80% of people surveyed considered their chances of being stopped by the police for BAC testing very low, while over 90% accepted the benefit of the law being enforced (*103*).

Pedestrians

Alcohol as a risk factor in pedestrian crashes has been well documented in high-income countries over several decades. Pedestrians impaired by alcohol, however, present a different order of risk to that of drinking drivers who pose more risks to themselves and others.

Clayton et al. established that for pedestrians there was a significantly higher risk of fatality relative to zero alcohol at BAC levels above 0.1 g/dl (*104*).

A review of Australian studies of alcohol involvement in pedestrian crashes showed that 20–30% of pedestrian casualties had a BAC level in excess of 0.15 g/dl, with alcohol involvement being greater among fatalities (*105*). Peden et al. (*98*) found that alcohol was a factor in over 61% of fatally-injured pedestrians in South Africa. A recent study in the United Kingdom concluded that 48% of pedestrians killed in road traffic collisions had been drinking, and that 39% of fatalities were over the legal BAC limit for driving (*106*). The proportion of male and female injured pedestrians consuming alcohol had increased by a third in the 16–19 years age group, when compared with findings from an earlier study conducted in 1985–1989 (*107*).

Medicinal and recreational drugs

While the contribution of alcohol to road crashes is much greater than that of any other drug, any medication or drug that affects the central nervous system has the potential to impair drivers (*108*). The effects, though, of both medicinal and recreational drugs on driving performance and crash involvement are much less well understood than those of alcohol, especially for low-income and middle-income countries. Determining the relationship between dose levels of drugs and increased crash risk is a complex matter. There exists a range of problems that make any interpretation of the relationship between drug levels (however measured) and driving safety extremely difficult, including the following:

- Most drugs, unlike alcohol, do not exhibit a simple relationship between drug blood-content and level of impairment (*109, 110*).
- Drugs within a particular category (e.g. antidepressants) can vary widely in their influence on behaviours, such as the distance a driver can brake in.
- Medically-impaired drivers may be safer driving with their drugs than without them, as in the case, for example, of schizophrenic patients with antipsychotic drugs (*111*).
- There are large individual differences in response to particular drugs.
- The short-term effects of certain drugs may differ from long-term effects (*112*).
- Many drugs are currently being used and several are often taken at the same time. Combinations of drugs may have synergistic effects (e.g. codeine and antipsychotic drugs with alcohol) or antagonistic effects. The number of possible interactions is great (*65, 113*).

Currently, there is no strong evidence that the use of drugs and driving constitutes a significant road crash risk. However, there is evidence for the increasing use among drivers of many psychoactive drugs, both medicinal and recreational, often in conjunction with alcohol (*114, 115*). This is an issue that needs urgent research.

Although studies support the notion that cannabis induces impairment (*109*), and in some countries there is a growing incidence of cannabis found in the blood of fatally-injured drivers, the evidence for its causal relationship with road traffic crashes remains undecided (*109, 116, 117*). A recent case–control study in France, though, found a higher prevalence of alcohol, cannabis and a combination of the two in blood samples from drivers involved in road crashes than in those from controls (*118*). A study in the United Kingdom also suggested a strong relationship between use of alcohol and cannabis together, and a clear reduction in driver capability following their use, compared with control data (*119*).

What is known suggests that drug use is a significant factor in some cultures but inadequate knowledge precludes quantifying the levels of risk at present. The availability and reliability of blood-screening procedures and confirmation tests for measuring alcohol and drug levels are problems for most low-income and middle-income countries. There is also the concern in high-income countries about screening for cannabis, since the substance can remain in the bloodstream for up to three weeks – hence making any attempt to link its use with driver impairment in a particular case exceptionally difficult.

Driver fatigue

Fatigue or sleepiness is associated with a range of factors (*120*) (see Table 3.5), including long-distance

TABLE 3.5

Factors that predispose a driver to fatigue			
Drivers at risk of fatigue	Temporal factors causing fatigue	Environmental factors in fatigue	Sleep-related factors
Young drivers (up to 25 years)	Driving between 02.00 and 05.00	Driving in remote areas with featureless terrain	Driving with sleep debt
Drivers over 50 years	More than 16 hours of wakefulness before trip	Monotonous roads	Driving with a sleep-related condition
Males	Long work period before trip	Main arterial roads	Driving when normally asleep
Shift workers	Long time since start of trip	Long-haul driving	Drivers disposed to nodding off
Those for whom driving is part of job	Irregular shift work before trip	Unexpected demands, breakdowns, etc.	Driving after poor-quality sleep
Those with medical conditions (such as narcolepsy)	Driving after successive nights of shift work	Extreme climatic conditions	
After consuming alcohol	Driving under time pressure	Driving an unfamiliar route	
Driving after inadequate rest and sleep	Some drivers are drowsy in the afternoon		

Source: reproduced from reference *120*, with minor editorial amendments, with the permission of the author.

driving, sleep deprivation and the disruption of circadian rhythms. Three high-risk groups have been
identified (*121*):

— young people, particularly males, aged
16–29 years;
— shift workers whose sleep is disrupted by
working at night or working long, irregular
hours;
— people with untreated sleep apnoea syn-
drome or narcolepsy.

Estimates of the proportion of car crashes attributable to driver sleepiness vary, depending on the
type of study and the quality of data. A population-
based case–control study in New Zealand found
that factors that substantially increased the risk of a
fatal crash or a crash with serious injuries were:

— driving while feeling sleepy;
— driving after less than five hours of sleep in
the preceding 24 hours;
— driving between 02:00 and 05:00.

The study concluded that a reduction in all three
of these behaviours could reduce the incidence of
crashes involving injury by up to 19% (*122*).

Surveys of commercial and public road transport in developing countries have revealed that
transport owners, in pursuit of increased profits,
frequently force their drivers to drive at excessive
speeds, to work unduly long hours and to work
when exhausted (*58, 59, 123*).

Studies by the National Transportation Safety
Board (NTSB) in the United States found that 52%
of 107 single-vehicle crashes involving heavy trucks
were fatigue-related and that in nearly 18% of the
cases, the drivers admitted to having fallen asleep.
The United States Department of Transportation's
investigations into fatigue in the 1990s showed that
fatigue was a factor in about 30% of fatal crashes
involving heavy commercial transport (*124–126*).

In Europe, studies have been less comprehensive,
and have often involved retrospective accounts that
were likely to underestimate the impact of fatigue.
These limitations notwithstanding, research from
some European countries suggests that driver
fatigue is a significant factor in approximately 20%
of commercial transport crashes. The results from
a range of surveys show that more than a half of

long-haul drivers have at some time fallen asleep at
the wheel (*127*).

Peak levels of fatigue-related crashes at night are
often 10 times higher than daytime levels. Research
in France on the working hours and habits of truck
drivers (*128*) showed that their risk of crashes
related to fatigue increased when:

— they were driving at night;
— the length of their working day had increased;
— they were working irregular hours.

Hand-held mobile telephones

The number of hand-held mobile telephones has
increased rapidly in many high-income countries
– in the United States, for example, from 500 000
in 1985 to over 120 million in 2001. Europe has
also seen sharp increases in their number (*129*).

The use of hand-held mobile telephones can
adversely affect driver behaviour – as regards physical
as well as perceptual and decision-making tasks. The
process of dialling influences a driver's ability to keep
to the course on the road (*130*). Results of studies on
distraction and mental load show that driver reaction
times are increased by 0.5–1.5 seconds when talking
into a mobile telephone (*131, 132*).

Studies have shown that driver performance is
particularly affected in maintaining the correct
lane position and the headway between two vehicles travelling one behind the other, in keeping to
an appropriate speed, and in judging and accepting
safe gaps in the traffic (*130, 131, 133, 134*). There is
also some evidence from studies that drivers who
use mobile telephones while driving face a risk of
a crash four times higher than those who do not
use them (*135*). Almost a half of drivers, though,
involved in a crash used a mobile telephone to
call for help (*135*). To date, at least 35 countries
or territories have banned the use of hand-held
mobile telephones while driving. While the use of
hands-free telephones can also distract drivers, the
current evidence suggests that the effect is less than
that for hand-held telephones (*129*).

Inadequate visibility

To see and be seen is a fundamental prerequisite
for the safety of all road users. Detailed studies

in Australia, Germany and Japan have shown that visual errors play a very important role in the cause of crashes (*136*).

In highly-motorized countries, inadequate visibility plays a key role in three types of crashes (*137*):

— a moving vehicle running into the rear or side of a slowly moving or stationary vehicle located ahead on the roadway, at night-time;
— angled collisions or head-on collisions in daytime;
— rear-end collisions in fog, in daytime and at night.

In low-income and middle-income countries, the phenomenon of pedestrians and vehicles not being properly visible is frequently a serious problem. In these places, there are fewer roads with adequate illumination and some may not be lit at all. In addition, it is more common for large numbers of bicycles and other vehicles to have no lights and for road space to be shared by fast-moving and slow-moving road users.

Cars and trucks

An analysis of crashes in the state of Victoria, Australia, suggests that not being sufficiently visible is a factor in 65% of crashes between cars and motorized two-wheelers and the sole cause in 21% of them (*138*). A meta-analysis of the effect of using daytime running lights found a 10–15% reduction in daytime crashes involving more than one party. A few countries currently require the fitting and use of daytime running lights (*139*).

Research in Germany has shown that nearly 5% of severe truck crashes can be traced back to poor visibility of the truck or its trailer at night. In these cases, car drivers failed to recognize trucks turning off the road, turning around or driving ahead of them (*140*).

A number of crashes involve drivers who fail to see other road users in the blind spots that exist in the area immediately around their vehicles. When larger vehicles such as trucks or buses are involved, these crashes frequently lead to serious injuries or even fatalities among vulnerable road users, such as pedestrians, cyclists or drivers of motorized two-wheelers (*141*).

Motorized two-wheelers

Motorized two-wheelers, because of their size and shape, are less easy to see than other motor vehicles and have poor visibility in daytime (*142*). A study in Malaysia found that most motorcycle crashes were in daytime and that around two-thirds of the riders involved had the right of way (*143*). Motorized two-wheelers that use daytime running lights have a crash rate about 10–29% lower than those that do not (*66, 144*).

Pedestrians and cyclists

In low-income countries, the mix of motorized and non-motorized traffic, together with frequent poor lighting, leads to a high risk for unprotected users if they are not seen by traffic. Lack of access to retro-reflective equipment, absence of bicycle lamp fitment, and use of darkly coloured bicycle helmets exacerbate already unsafe conditions. A review of European in-depth research found that one third of pedestrian casualties had difficulty in seeing the striking vehicle. Similarly, two fifths of drivers had difficulty in seeing the pedestrian (*63*). The more conspicuous a particular motor vehicle is to all other road users, and the more visible the other road users are to the particular driver, then the greater the opportunity of avoiding a collision. More than 30% of bicycle crashes in the Netherlands occurring at night or in twilight could have been avoided, it is estimated, if bicycle lighting had been used (*145*).

Road-related factors

Road crashes tend not to be evenly distributed throughout the network. They occur in clusters at single sites, along particular sections of road, or scattered across whole residential neighbourhoods, especially in areas of social deprivation (*146*). While road engineering can greatly help in reducing the frequency and severity of road traffic crashes, poor engineering can contribute to crashes. The road network has an effect on crash risk because it determines how road users perceive their environment and provides instructions for road users, through signs and traffic controls, on what they should be doing. Many traffic management and road safety engineering measures work through their influence on human behaviour (*6*).

Negative road engineering factors include those where a road defect directly triggers a crash, where some element of the road environment misleads a road user and thereby creates error, or where some feasible physical alteration to the road that would have made the crash less likely has not been made (*147*).

In the planning, design and maintenance of the road network, four particular elements affecting road safety have been identified (*148*). These elements are:

— safety-awareness in the planning of new road networks;
— the incorporation of safety features in the design of new roads;
— safety improvements to existing roads;
— remedial action at high-risk crash sites.

The absence of any of these elements, discussed below, are risk factors for crashes.

Inattention to safety in planning new road networks

As already mentioned, crash risks in road networks are frequently increased by the existence of unnecessary motorized travel, by policies encouraging travel by less safe modes, and by the creation of unsafe mixes of travel (*5*).

Specific situations related to road planning that are risk factors for crashes include (*5, 148*):

— through-traffic passing through residential areas;
— conflicts between pedestrians and vehicles near schools located on busy roads;
— lack of segregation of pedestrians and high-speed traffic;
— lack of median barriers to prevent dangerous overtaking on single-carriageway roads;
— lack of barriers to prevent pedestrian access onto high-speed dual-carriageway roads.

The growth in urbanization and in the number of motorized vehicles in many low-income and middle-income countries has not been accompanied by adequate attention to road design.

Inattention to safety in designing roads

Where road layouts are self-explanatory to their users – through the use of markings, signs and physically self-enforcing measures to reduce speed – engineering can have a beneficial influence on behaviour. Engineering design, though, can often have negative influences on behaviour – when there is incompatibility between the function of the roads, their layout and their use, this creates risk for road users.

Uncertainty among road users about the layout of roads – through the absence of clear and unambiguous markings and signs – is a particular risk factor for crashes. Similarly, the lack of self-enforcing measures to reduce speed will increase the risk.

Straight, unmarked single-carriageway roads encourage drivers to speed. Other risk factors are the poor design and control of junctions and insufficient lighting.

Safety defects in existing roads

Defects contributing to crash risk can appear in road designs, especially if they have not been subject to a safety audit by experienced safety personnel. Such defects are frequently caused by the poor design of junctions or by design that allows for large differences in the speed and the mass of vehicles and in the direction of travel.

Bad road surface conditions are a particular risk factor for users of motorized two-wheelers. Often, where there is no safety impact study to assess the effects of a new road scheme on the existing network, a new road scheme can have an adverse impact on large areas.

Lack of remedial action at high-risk crash sites

Large numbers of high-risk crash sites exist everywhere, located either at isolated spots or grouped along particular stretches of road. Many of them are well-known and documented. Some 145 dangerous locations, for example, have been identified on Kenya's main rural road network (*149*). If such sites are not dealt with, promptly and systematically, there will be a great risk of further crashes.

A survey of 12 European Union countries found that many of them lacked comprehensive remedial programmes for high-risk sites (*147*). The survey showed that:

— only seven countries reported having a formal policy;

— only six had national guidelines or manuals;

— only five reported taking specific steps to stimulate remedial schemes;

— only three reported having a separate national budget;

— only three reported that evaluations were standard practice in applying remedial schemes.

Vehicle-related risk factors

While vehicle design can have considerable influence on crash injuries, its contribution to crashes, through vehicle defects, is generally around 3% in high-income countries (*150*), about 5% in Kenya (*4*) and 3% in South Africa (*151*).

Though periodic vehicle inspections have not been found useful in reducing injury crashes, inspections and checks for overloading and safety-related maintenance for larger commercial vehicles and buses could be important for vehicles more than 12 years old (*152*).

While there is in general no evidence that periodic motor vehicle inspections reduce crash rates, the exception is in the field of commercial vehicles, where defective brakes on large trucks have been shown to be a risk factor (*153*).

Risk factors influencing injury severity

Well-established risk factors that contribute to the severity of a crash include:

— inadequate in-vehicle crash protection;

— inadequate roadside protection;

— the non-use of protective devices in vehicles;

— the non-use of protective crash helmets;

— excessive and inappropriate speed;

— the presence of alcohol.

Lack of in-vehicle crash protection

In the past decade, the crashworthiness of private cars for their occupants has improved considerably in many high-income countries, though there is considerable room for further improvement (*53, 71, 154, 155*).

In low-income countries, the regulation of motor vehicle safety standards is not as systematic as in high-income countries. Many engineering advances that are found in vehicles available in high-income countries are not standard fittings in vehicles in low-income countries (*4*). In addition, the majority of road casualties in low-income countries occur outside the car, with those affected being pedestrians, cyclists, motorized two-wheeled vehicle riders or passengers in buses and trucks. As yet, there are no requirements to protect vulnerable road users by means of crash-worthy designs for the fronts of cars or buses (*61*).

Car occupants

The main injury risks for car occupants arise from the way vehicles interact with each other and with the roadside in frontal and side-impact crashes. In fatal and serious crashes, head, chest and abdominal injuries are predominant. Among injuries that cause disablement, those to the legs and neck are important. Determinants for the degree of severity of injuries include:

— contact by occupant with the car's interior, exacerbated by intrusion into the passenger compartment caused by the colliding vehicle or object;

— mismatch in terms of size and weight between vehicles involved in a crash;

— ejection from the vehicle;

— inadequate vehicle safety standards.

The European Commission has stated that if all cars were designed to be equal in standard to the best car currently available in each class, then an estimated 50% of all fatal and disabling injuries could be avoided (*53*).

The relationship between vehicle age and risk of a car crash with injury has recently been investigated. The study showed that occupants in cars manufactured before 1984 have approximately three times the risk of a car crash injury compared with occupants of newer cars (*156*).

Pedestrians

Crashes between vehicles and pedestrians are responsible for more than a third of all traffic-related deaths and injuries worldwide (*62*). Compared with vehicle occupant casualties, pedestrians sustain more multiple injuries, with higher injury severity scores and higher mortality rates (*157*).

Research in Europe suggests that two thirds of all fatally-injured pedestrians are hit by the front of a car; 11% are hit by other parts of a car. Impacts with all other types of vehicle account for the remaining 23% of pedestrian fatalities (*154*). In many low-income and middle-income countries, buses and trucks are also a major source of injury through impact for pedestrians, bicyclists and motorized two-wheeler riders. In India, in the cities and on rural highways, buses and trucks are involved in more than 50% of the crashes affecting pedestrians (*158*). The distribution of different vehicle types involved in pedestrian crashes in Ghana, shown in Table 3.6, is fairly typical for low-income countries. In Ghana, car-to-pedestrian impacts are the leading cause of pedestrian death and injury, followed by collisions of buses or minibuses with pedestrians.

TABLE 3.6

Frequency of involvement of different vehicles in pedestrian crashes and fatalities in Ghana, 1998–2000

Vehicle type	Percentage involvement in all crashes	Percentage involvement in fatal crashes
Cars/taxis	54.0	37.8
Bicycle	5.2	0.8
Motorcycle	2.8	2.1
Bus/minibus	23.4	31.8
Heavy goods vehicle	7.3	18.6
Pick-up trucks	6.4	7.6
Others	0.9	1.3

Source: reproduced from reference *56*, with the permission of the publisher.

There are usually two phases in car-to-pedestrian collisions. The first and most severe phase consists of multiple impacts with different parts of the car front. The second phase is contact with the road surface, where injuries are generally minor (*159*).

The most frequent causes of serious and fatal pedestrian injuries in collisions with cars stem from impacts between (*160*):

— the head of the pedestrian and the whole area of the car bonnet top and windscreen frame;
— the pelvis or the abdomen of adults and the bonnet edge;
— the abdomen or chest of children or the head of small children and the bonnet edge;
— the legs and the car bumper.

In general, lower-limb trauma is the most common form of pedestrian injury, while head injury is responsible for most pedestrian fatalities (*62*).

Results from both the Australian and the European New Car Assessment Programmes, using four performance tests, indicate that, in general, the new cars tested did not provide protection for pedestrians and cyclists (*161, 162*).

Users of motorized two-wheelers

Hospital studies in Thailand show that 75–80% of road casualties and 70–90% of road deaths are among motorized two-wheeler users (*15*).

Motorized two-wheeler users tend to sustain multiple injuries, including to the head, chest and legs. The majority of the fatal injuries are to the head. Lower-leg injuries – either from direct contact with the impacting vehicle or as a result of being crushed – contribute substantially to morbidity (*163*). A Malaysian study found that leg injuries usually required a longer period of inpatient stay than other non-fatal injuries (*164*).

Considerable research has been conducted in Europe to identify effective leg protection for motorized two-wheeler riders and to develop suitable air bags to protect riders in case of a frontal impact (*165*).

Bus and truck occupants

Buses with passengers, minibuses and trucks are frequently involved in crashes in low-income countries. The use of open-backed vehicles for transporting passengers in rural areas is widespread and risks ejecting passengers (*166*). In New Delhi, India, around two thirds of crashes involve buses or trucks (*5*).

In many low-income and middle-income countries, second-hand trucks and buses are imported without the crash-protective features – such as occupant restraints – that are present in high-income countries. Such vehicles have a poor crashworthiness performance, and also poor stability when fully laden or overloaded, as they frequently are.

The urban centres of low-income and middle-income countries typically contain a great mix of vehicles. Incompatibility of size between different classes of road vehicles is a major risk factor, especially in impacts between cars and large trucks. The power of the larger vehicle – its mass, geometry and structural properties – increases rates of injury and death many times compared with an equivalent car-to-car crash (71, 167).

Safer bus and truck fronts have been identified as an urgent need (71, 141, 168). A study in New Delhi showed that of 359 crashes involving trucks, 55% also involved vulnerable road users. Impacts between the fronts of trucks and pedestrians resulted in severe leg injuries at 25 km/h. At 35 km/h the head sustained severe injuries, as did the chest at 45 km/h. Contact with bumpers resulted in pelvic injury (141).

Non-use of crash helmets by two-wheeled vehicle users

Users of motorized two-wheelers

The main risk factor for motorized two-wheeler users is the non-use of crash helmets. Use of helmets has been shown to reduce fatal and serious head injuries by between 20% and 45% and to be the most successful approach for preventing injury among motorized two-wheeler riders (169).

Head trauma is the main cause of death and morbidity in motorized two-wheeler users, contributing to around 75% of motorized two-wheeler deaths in European countries (170). Fatal head injury resulting from crashes is estimated to account for 55–88% of motorized two-wheeler rider deaths in Malaysia (171). Substantial growths in motorized two-wheeler use in low-income and middle-income countries are being accompanied by an increase in head injuries.

Kulanthayan et al. (172) found that non-helmeted motorized two-wheeler users were three times more likely to sustain head injuries in a crash than those wearing helmets. A study of crash victims admitted to a neurosurgery ward in New Delhi, India showed that riders who used any type of helmet with some protective padding benefited (94). Helmet use varies from slightly over zero in some low-income countries to almost 100% in places where laws on helmet use are effectively enforced. Helmets constructed in some low-income and middle-income countries are not always appropriately designed. In some countries, such as Malaysia, special exemptions from wearing a helmet are given to certain religious groups, such as Sikhs. In several low-income countries, helmet use has been found to be lower at night (173, 174). Though the wearing of helmets has generally been widespread in most high-income countries, there is some evidence of a decline. In the United States, for example, helmet use fell sharply to 58% in 2002 from 71% recorded two years previously (175).

Studies in low-income countries have found that more than half of adult motorized two-wheeler riders do not wear their helmets properly secured (172, 176). Child passengers rarely wear helmets and if helmets are used at all they are likely to be adult helmets, providing almost no protection (177). A study in California, United States, found that nearly half of motorcyclists used non-standard helmets and that these riders incurred more frequent head injuries than those who wore either standard helmets or no helmets at all (178).

Bicycle helmets

Admissions to hospital and deaths from bicycle-related trauma are usually due to head injury (179). Bicycle helmets reduce the risk of head and brain injuries by between 63% and 88% (180–182).

A meta-analysis of studies on the benefits of bicycle helmets found that wearing a helmet had an odds-ratio efficacy of 0.40, 0.42, 0.53 and 0.27 for head, brain, facial and fatal injuries, respectively (183).

Several countries have introduced legislation on bicycle helmet wearing, including Australia, New Zealand, Sweden and the United States. In countries which do not require the use of helmets by law, the wearing rate is normally less than 10%

(*184*). Rates of helmet use tend to be higher among younger children, as opposed to teenagers and adults.

Non-use of seat-belts and child restraints in motor vehicles

Failure to use seat-belts is a major risk factor for vehicle occupants. The most frequent and most serious injuries occurring in frontal impacts to occupants unrestrained by seat-belts are to the head (*185*). The effectiveness of seat-belts depends upon the type and severity of the crash and the seating position of the occupant. The benefits of seat-belts in terms of injury reduction and their effectiveness in different types of impacts are set out in Tables 3.7 and 3.8.

Crash research in various countries has found that rates of seat-belt wearing are substantially lower in fatal collisions than the general average rate. For example, while the overall proportion of occupants wearing seat-belts in traffic is around 90%, only around 55% of drivers in fatal crashes in Finland wore seat-belts (*189*), and about 35% in Sweden (*190*).

While seat-belts may cause injuries, these are, typically, minor abrasions and bruising to the chest and abdomen, and without the seat-belts the injuries would have been far more severe (*191*). The effectiveness of front seat-belts in a frontal collision is reduced by the rear loading caused by unrestrained passengers in the back seat. This phenomenon of rear loading can cause severe chest injuries to the occupants of front seats. It can also occur when there

TABLE 3.7

Injury reduction benefits of seat-belts for car drivers and front-seat passengers

Year	Reference	Injury reducing effect (%)		
		Fatal collisions	Moderate and severe injuries	All severities
1976	Griffith et al.	41		
1984	Hobbs & Mills		65	
1986	Department of Transport, USA			40–50
1987	Malliaris & Digges	50 (drivers) 40 (front-seat passengers)		
1987	Evans	41		
1987	Campbell	65 (drivers) 54 (front-seat passengers)	51–52 (drivers) 43–44 (front-seat passengers)	
1996	National Highway Traffic Safety Administration, USA		48	
1996	Cooperative Crash Injury Study, UK (unpublished)		53	
2003	Cummings et al.	61		
	Effectiveness range	40–65	43–65	40–50

Source: reproduced from references *186, 187.*

TABLE 3.8

Injury reduction effects of seat-belts for various types of car crash

Crash type	Proportion of all crashes (%)	Driver seat-belt effectiveness in different crash types (%)
Frontal	59	43
Struck side	14	27
Non-struck side	9	39
Rear	5	49
Roll-over	14	77

Source: reproduced from reference *188*, with the permission of the publisher.

is unrestrained luggage on the rear seats. Earlier concerns that seat-belt use would lead routinely to death by entrapment or to problems in pregnancy, or would encourage drivers to take greater risks, have not been borne out by empirical evidence (*185, 192–194*).

Extent of the problem

Rates of seat-belt use vary greatly among different countries, depending upon the existence of laws mandating their fitting and use, and the degree to which those laws are enforced. In many low-income countries, there is no requirement for belts to be fitted in motor vehicles or to be used. Despite legislation, though, the extent of non-use remains significant in highly-motorized countries, with low rates of front seat-belt wearing in some places and generally low rates of rear seat-belt wearing. In the United States, front seat-belt use was reported in 2002 as 75%, compared with 58% in 1994 (175). In European Union countries in the mid-1990s, wearing rates of front seat-belts ranged between 52% and 92%, and those of rear seat-belts between 9% and 80% (186).

In the Republic of Korea, rates of seat-belt usage rose sharply among drivers, from 23% in late 2000 to 98% in August 2001, following a national campaign of police enforcement together with publicity and a doubling of the fine for non-use (195). In many other places, including some eastern European countries and parts of Central and South America, usage rates are generally much lower. In Argentina, for instance, front seat-belt use is around 26% in the capital Buenos Aires and 58% on national highways (196).

A survey in Kenya found that of over 200 road crash survivors only 1% reported seat-belt use, leading the authors of the study to conclude that "the demand for seat-belts has yet to become part of the culture in Kenya" (59).

In some countries, usage among drivers tends to be high on motorways but low in urban areas. Young male drivers have been found to use their safety belts less often than other groups and are also more often involved in crashes (197).

Child restraints

Methods of restraining children in motor vehicles, and in particular the use of child safety seats, vary within and between countries. In high-income countries, usage rates of child restraints tend to be high – about 90% in Australia and 86% in the United States. In car travel in low-income countries, though, their use is rare.

Child restraints work in the same way as adult seat-belts. Rear-facing seats have been shown to be particularly effective (see Table 3.9). When travel-

ling rearwards, the forces from a sudden deceleration will be distributed over the child's body and head in an optimal way, which markedly increases effectiveness.

TABLE 3.9

Injury reduction benefits of child restraints

Type of restraint	All injuries (%)	Severe injuries (%)
Rearward facing	76	92
Forward facing	34	60

Source: reproduced from reference 186, with the permission of the publisher.

In terms of preventing fatalities, the use of safety seats for children travelling in cars offers a very high level of protection. It has been shown to reduce infant deaths in cars by approximately 71% and deaths of small children by 54% (198). Nevertheless even when restrained, children in cars face a particular risk from side impacts. A study in Sweden showed that approximately 50% of fatally-injured children aged up to 3 years had been involved in side impact collisions (199). The European New Car Assessment Programme has also shown that current restraints, when fitted in cars, do not fully constrain the movement of the child's head and prevent contact with the car's interior (154).

Air bags

Driver air bags are designed to provide protection for belted and unbelted occupants in frontal crashes. Estimates of their effectiveness in reducing driver deaths in purely frontal crashes range from 22% to 29% (187, 200–202).

The potential hazard of combining air bags with rear-facing child safety seats in the front seat was first reported in 1974 by Aldman et al. (203), and more recently by Anund (204) and Weber (205). In the United States, there have been many cases of fatally injured and severely injured children where the injuries – attributed to air bags that inflated during low-speed car crashes – might not otherwise have been sustained. Given the popularity of rear-facing child safety seats in Europe and the almost universal practice in high-income countries of fitting air bags on the front passenger side of the vehicle, action has recently been taken in some places to legislate for the provision of warning labels in cars and of automatic sensors that can detect the presence of occupants seated in front of the air bag.

Studies have shown that there is a substantial amount of incorrect use of both adult seat-belts and child restraints, which markedly lessens their potential to reduce injury (*206, 207*).

Roadside objects

Impacts between vehicles leaving the road and solid roadside objects such as trees, poles and road signs are a major road safety problem worldwide. According to research in Australia and several European Union countries, roadside hazards contribute to between 18% and 42% of fatal crashes (*208, 209*).

These collisions are usually single-vehicle crashes and frequently involve young drivers, excess or inappropriate speed, the use of alcohol or driver fatigue. Another problem related to impacts with objects off the road is the occurrence of crashes caused by restricted visibility, due to the poor siting of these objects.

The linkages between vehicle crash protection and roadside crash protection need to be strengthened. For example, cars do not provide protection for occupants in head-on collisions at speeds above 60–70 km/h (or even lower limits with other types of impact), although many cars travel at these and higher speeds. For this reason, the road environment needs to be designed so as to eliminate head-on collisions – into trees, poles and other rigid objects – at high speeds, where the car itself cannot offer sufficient protection. Cars, roads and other aspects of the traffic system must be designed in a mutually-linked way (*155*).

Risk factors influencing post-crash injury outcome

Studies worldwide have shown that death was potentially preventable in a large proportion of those who died as a result of road crashes before they reached hospital (*210, 211*).

A review of European studies of mortality in road traffic concluded that about 50% of deaths from road collisions occurred within a few min-

utes at the scene of the crash, or else on the way to a hospital but before arrival there. For those patients taken to hospital, the data suggest that comparatively few deaths, only about 15%, occur between one and four hours after the incident, while around 35% occur after four hours. The time between the incident and death varies considerably between patients and between countries (*212*).

A comparative study of mortality among seriously injured patients across a range of countries found that for low-income and middle-income countries, the vast majority of deaths occurred in the pre-hospital phase (see Table 3.10). The study also showed clearly that the probability of dying increased as the socioeconomic level of the victim decreased (*213*). Morbidity outcomes are also influenced by factors related to post-impact care. A study in the United Kingdom, for instance, suggested that 12% of patients who had sustained serious skeletal trauma went on to experience significant disability that was preventable (*214*).

TABLE 3.10

Proportion of road deaths by setting in three cities

Setting	Kumasi, Ghana (%)	Monterrey, Mexico (%)	Seattle, USA (%)
Pre-hospital	81	72	59
Emergency room	5	21	18
Hospital ward	14	7	23

Source: reference *213*.

In the case of major injuries, the potential help towards recovery that survivors can receive can be viewed as a chain with several links (*212*):

— actions, or self-help, at the scene of the crash, by the victims themselves, or more frequently by bystanders;
— access to the emergency medical system;
— help provided by rescuers of the emergency services;
— delivery of medical care before arrival at the hospital;
— hospital trauma care;
— rehabilitative psychosocial care.

Pre-hospital factors

Weak public health infrastructure in many low-income and middle-income countries is a major risk factor. In high-income countries, the pre-hospital risk factors are not so pronounced, but where they exist, are associated with the need to improve the existing elements of post-impact care. In most highly-motorized countries, the large volume of traffic and the high incidence of mobile telephones usually lead to the early alerting of the medical services about a crash. However, in low-income countries, most of the population does not have access to even the most basic form of emergency medical service. Evacuation and transport to hospital is more often carried out by bystanders, relatives, commercial vehicles or the police (215). An African study found that the police and hospital ambulances evacuated only 5.5% and 2.9%, respectively, of crash victims in Kenya (216).

Research in the United States has shown that the transport by ambulance can be a risk, as a result of the high speeds of travel and the frequent lack of available restraint. Compared with police cars and fire trucks, ambulances experience the greatest proportion of fatal crashes in which occupants are killed as well as the greatest proportion of crashes in which occupants are injured (217).

In low-income countries, many victims do not possess social security, health cover or life insurance and therefore lack access to hospital care (59, 60). In a study carried out in Ghana, overall hospital use was found to be very low, with only 27% of all injured people using hospital services. Among those with severe injuries, only 60% of urban casualties and 38% of rural casualties received hospital care (210).

Hospital care factors

Lack of trained expertise in trauma care

Trauma treatment in high-income countries is usually seen as a chain of care performed by well-trained practitioners, even if many of its elements have room for improvement (212, 213). In low-income countries, the post-impact chain of care is often delivered by personnel lacking formal training. A study in Mexico showed that this was the case throughout much of the emergency medical services (218). In Ghana, a study of 11 rural hospitals that received large numbers of road traffic casualties was staffed exclusively by general practitioners without trauma training (210).

A further risk factor in low-income countries is the lack of sufficient numbers of formally trained surgeons. In the late 1980s, it was estimated there were 50 surgeons per 100 000 people in the United States, as opposed to only 7 per 100 000 in Latin America and 0.5 per 100 000 in Africa (219).

A study of 2000 trauma admissions in the main hospital in Kumasi, Ghana, found a mean 12-hour delay before the start of emergency surgery as well as low rates of usage of key equipment, despite its availability (210).

Lack of equipment

Adequate trauma care requires a range of medical specialities and equipment, as well as appropriate logistic support to ensure that the equipment and other specialities are available to the patient on arrival. In reality, delays are substantial and frequent, introducing avoidable risks of complications.

In the study of 11 Ghanaian hospitals, essential low-cost and reusable equipment was lacking – because of poor organization rather than the cost. For example, no hospital had chest tubes and only four had equipment to ensure a patent airway (210). In Kenya, in a survey of hospital administrators, only 40% of the health facilities – both outpatient and inpatient services – were reported to be well prepared and have key supplies available (216).

Conclusion

Analysis of available crash data and other road traffic research show that while the main road safety problems experienced in various parts of the world often differ in quality and quantity, they have many characteristics in common. The dominant, common characteristics of the risks associated with road traffic are as follows:

- Unnecessary travel, the choice of less safe travel modes and routes, and unsafe mixes of traffic all lead to increased risk.

- The design of roads and road networks is an important factor. Exposure to risk is increased significantly by road networks failing to route heavy traffic around populated areas or to separate pedestrians from motorized traffic.
- Excess and inappropriate speed is widespread and may contribute to around 30% of road traffic crashes and deaths. In collisions at 80 km/h, car occupants run a 20 times higher risk of being killed than at 30 km/h. Pedestrians have a 90% chance of surviving car crashes at 30 km/h or below, but less than a 50% chance of surviving impacts at 45 km/h or above.
- Impairment by alcohol continues to contribute to crash injury and increases the risk. All non-zero BAC levels carry more risk than zero BAC, and crash risk starts to rise sharply at levels of 0.04 g/dl. Legal BAC limits set at 0.10 g/dl allow three times more risk than limits set at 0.05 g/dl; at 0.08 g/dl, the risk is twice as much as that at 0.05 g/dl.
- Young novice drivers are at increased risk of crash injury; the risk among teenage drivers is higher than among any other comparable age group. Excess or inappropriate speed is a common contributory factor in crashes involving young drivers.
- Pedestrians, cyclists and motorized two-wheeler users bear a disproportionate share of the global road injury burden and are all at high risk of crash injury.
- For all road users, the risk of crash injury is increased by failing to see and failing to be seen. If daytime running lights were fitted and used, almost a third of all motorized two-wheeler crashes involving lack of visibility could be avoided; in the case of cars, more than 10% of such crashes could be avoided.
- The non-use of seat-belts and child restraints more than doubles the risk of serious and fatal injury, as does the non-use of bicycle helmets. Similarly, the non-use of crash helmets by motorized two-wheeler users almost doubles their risk of serious or fatal head injury.

- Crash analysis shows that the majority of pedestrian fatalities involve impact with unprotective car fronts. If all cars were designed to provide protection equivalent to that of the best car in the same class, an estimated half of all fatal and disabling injuries to car occupants would be avoided. Roadside design and the positioning of roadside objects play key roles in determining crash injury, as well as influencing the behaviour of road users.
- Inadequate post-crash care is a major problem in many places. The availability and quality of such care has a substantial effect on whether a road traffic injury leads to subsequent death or disability.

The availability in low-income countries of data on road traffic crashes is often basic. For a proper understanding of the risk factors predominating in local settings, more investment for systematic, independent and high-quality research is needed, particularly from high-income countries. Such worldwide research into the causes of crashes and crash injury is essential for achieving safer traffic systems.

References

1. Tingvall C. The Zero Vision. In: van Holst H, Nygren A, Thord R, eds. *Transportation, traffic safety and health: the new mobility. Proceedings of the 1st International Conference, Gothenburg, Sweden, 1995.* Berlin, Springer-Verlag, 1995:35–57.

2. Rumar K. *Transport safety visions, targets and strategies: beyond 2000.* Brussels, European Transport Safety Council, 1999 (1st European Transport Safety Lecture) (http://www.etsc.be/eve.htm, accessed 30 October 2003).

3. MacKay GM. Some features of road trauma in developing countries. In: *Proceedings of the International Association for Accident and Traffic Medicine Conference, Mexico, DF, September 1983.* Stockholm, International Association for Accident and Traffic Medicine, 1983:21–25.

4. Odero W, Garner P, Zwi AB. Road traffic injuries in developing countries: a comprehensive review of epidemiological studies. *Tropical Medicine and International Health,* 1997, 2:445–460.

5. Mohan D, Tiwari G. Road safety in low-income countries: issues and concerns regarding technology transfer from high-income countries. In: *Reflections on the transfer of traffic safety knowledge to motorising nations*. Melbourne, Global Traffic Safety Trust, 1998:27–56.

6. Ogden KW. *Safer roads: a guide to road safety engineering*. Melbourne, Ashgate Publishing Ltd, 1996.

7. Whitelegg J. *A comparison of road traffic accidents and injuries in Köln and Manchester. Final Report*. Dortmund, Institut für Stadt- und Landentwicklungsforschung des Landes Nordrhein-Westphalen, 1988.

8. Smeed R. Some statistical aspects of road safety research. *Journal of the Royal Statistical Society,* 1949, 112(Series A):1–34.

9. Tunali O. The billion-car accident waiting to happen. *World Watch*, 1996, 9:24–39.

10. Lowe MD. *Alternatives to the automobiles: transport for livable cities*. Washington, DC, World Watch Institute, 1990 (World Watch Paper No. 98).

11. Vasconcellos EA. *Urban transport, environment and equity: the case for developing countries*. London, Earthscan Publications, 2001.

12. Wintemute GJ. Is motor vehicle-related mortality a disease of development? *Accident Analysis and Prevention*, 1985, 17:223–237.

13. Sweedler BM. The worldwide decline in drinking and driving. In: Kloeden CN, McLean AJ, eds. *Proceedings of the 13th International Conference on Alcohol, Drugs and Traffic Safety, Adelaide, 13–18 August 1995*. Adelaide, Road Accident Research Unit, 1995.

14. Kopits E, Cropper M. *Traffic fatalities and economic growth*. Washington, DC, The World Bank, 2003 (Policy Research Working Paper No. 3035).

15. Suriyawongpaisal P, Kanchanusut S. Road traffic injuries in Thailand: trends, selected underlying determinants and status of intervention. *Injury Control and Safety Promotion,* 2003, 10:95–104.

16. Ghaffar A et al. Injuries in Pakistan: directions for future health policy. *Health Policy and Planning*, 1999, 14:11–17.

17. Winston FK et al. The carnage wrought by major economic change: ecological study of traffic-related mortality and the re-unification of Germany. *British Medical Journal,* 1999, 318: 1647–1650.

18. Mikulik J. Relation among accident development and political/social changes. In: *Joint Economic Commission for Africa/Organisation for Economic Co-operation and Development. Third African road safety congress. Compendium of papers, volume 1. 14–17 April 1997, Pretoria, South Africa*. Addis Ababa, Economic Commission for Africa, 1997:104–117.

19. Roberts I, Crombie I. Child pedestrian deaths: sensitivity to traffic volume – evidence from the USA. *Journal of Epidemiology and Community Health*, 1995, 49:186–188.

20. Roberts I, Marshall R, Norton R. Child pedestrian mortality and traffic volume in New Zealand. *British Medical Journal,* 1992, 305:283.

21. *Report of the Regional Director to the Regional Committee for the Western Pacific*. Manila, World Health Organization Regional Office for the Western Pacific, 2003.

22. Chiu W et al. The effect of the Taiwan motorcycle helmet use law on head injuries. *American Journal of Public Health*, 2000, 90:793–796.

23. *Road accidents in Great Britain: the casualty report*. London, Department for Transport, 2001.

24. Varghese M. Analysis of 198 medical-legal records of road traffic accident victims treated in a Delhi hospital. *Journal of Traffic Medicine*, 1990, 18:280.

25. Salifu M. Urban pedestrian accidents in Ghana. *Research Journal of the International Association of Traffic and Safety Sciences*, 1996, 20:131–140.

26. Khayesi M. Liveable streets for pedestrians in Nairobi: the challenge of road traffic accidents. In: Whitelegg J, Haq G, eds. *The Earthscan reader on world transport policy and practice*. London, Earthscan Publications, 2003:35–41.

27. Hakamies-Blomqvist L. *Ageing Europe: the challenges and opportunities for transport safety* [The 5th European Transport Safety Lecture]. Brussels, European Transport Safety Council, 2003 (http://www.etsc.be/eve.htm, accessed 17 November 2003).

28. *Report on transport and ageing of the population*. Paris, European Conference of Ministers of Transport, Council of Ministers, 2001 (CEMT/CM(2001)16) (http://www1.oecd.org/cem/

topics/council/cmpdf/2001/CM0116e.pdf, accessed 17 November 2003).

29. Litman T. *If health matters: integrating public health objectives in transportation planning.* Victoria, BC, Victoria Transport Policy Institute, 2003.

30. Khayesi M. The need for an integrated road safety programme for the city of Nairobi, Kenya. In: Freeman P, Jamet C, eds. *Urban transport policy: a sustainable development tool. Proceedings of the 8th CODATU International Conference, Cape Town, 21–25 September 1998.* Rotterdam, AA Balkema Publishers, 1998:579–582.

31. Tiwari G. Traffic flow and safety: need for new models for heterogeneous traffic. In: Mohan D, Tiwari G, eds. *Injury prevention and control.* London, Taylor and Francis, 2000:71–88.

32. Koornstra MK, ed. *Transport safety performance in the EU.* Brussels, European Transport Safety Council, Transport Accident Statistics Working Party, 2003 (http://www.etsc.be/rep.htm, accessed 17 November 2003).

33. Miller T et al. Is it safest to travel by bicycle, car or big truck? *Journal of Crash Prevention and Injury Control,* 1999, 1:25–34.

34. Allsop R. *Road safety: Britain in Europe.* London, Parliamentary Advisory Council for Transport Safety, 2001 (http://www.pacts.org.uk/richardslecture.htm, accessed 30 October 2003).

35. *Impacts monitoring first annual report.* London, Transport for London, 2003.

36. *Towards the year 2010: monitoring casualties in Greater London.* London, Transport for London, London Accident Analysis Unit, 2003.

37. Allsop RE ed. *Reducing traffic injuries from inappropriate speed.* Brussels, European Transport Safety Council, 1995.

38. Nilsson G. *The effects of speed limits on traffic accidents in Sweden.* Sartryck, Swedish National Road and Transport Research Institute, 1982.

39. Andersson G, Nilsson G. *Speed management in Sweden.* Linköping, Swedish National Road and Transport Research Institute, 1997.

40. Finch DJ et al. *Speed, speed limits and accidents.* Crowthorne, Transport Research Laboratory, 1994 (Project Report 58).

41. Taylor MC, Lynam DA, Baruya A. *The effects of drivers' speed on the frequency of road accidents.* Crowthorne, Transport Research Laboratory, 2000 (TRL Report 421).

42. Taylor MC, Baruya A, Kennedy JV. *The relationship between speed and accidents on rural single-carriageway roads.* Crowthorne, Transport Research Laboratory, 2002 (TRL Report 511).

43. Elvik R, Mysen AB, Vaa T. *Trafikksikkerhetshåndbok, tredje utgave [Handbook of traffic safety, 3rd ed.].* Oslo, Institute of Transport Economics, 1997.

44. Munden JM. *The relation between a driver's speed and his accident rate.* Crowthorne, Road Research Laboratory, 1967 (RRL Report LR 88).

45. McLean J, Kloeden C. Alcohol, travelling speed and the risk of crash involvement. In: Mayhew DR, Dussault C, eds. *Proceedings of the 16th International Conference on Alcohol, Drugs and Traffic Safety, Montreal, 4–9 August 2002.* Montreal, Société de l'assurance automobile du Québec, 2002:73–79 (http://www.saaq.gouv.qc.ca/t2002/actes/pdf/(07a).pdf, accessed 17 November 2003).

46. Mackay M, Hassan AM. Age and gender effects on injury outcome for restrained occupants in frontal crashes. In: *Proceedings of the Association for the Advancement of Automotive Medicine Conference.* Chicago, IL, Association for the Advancement of Automotive Medecine, 2000:75–92.

47. Hobbs CA, Mills PJ. *Injury probability for car occupants in frontal and side impacts.* Crowthorne, Transport Research Laboratory, 1984 (TRL Report 1124).

48. *IIHS Facts: 55 speed limit.* Arlington, VA, Insurance Institute for Highway Safety, 1987.

49. Pasanen E. *Ajonopeudet ja jalankulkijan turvallisuus [Driving speeds and pedestrian safety].* Espoo, Teknillinen korkeakoulu, Liikennetekniikka, 1991.

50. Ashton SJ, Mackay GM. Benefits from changes in vehicle exterior design. In: *Proceedings of the Society of Automotive Engineers.* Detroit, MI, Society of Automotive Engineers, 1983:255–264 (Publication No. 121).

51. Ashton SJ, Mackay GM. Car design for pedestrian injury minimisation. In: *Proceedings of the Seventh Experimental Safety of Vehicles Conference, Paris, 5–8 June 1979.* Washington, DC, National Highway Traffic Safety Administration, 1979:630–640.

52. Leaf WA, Preusser DF. *Literature review on vehicle travel speeds and pedestrian injuries.* Washington, DC, National Highway Traffic Safety Administration, 1999 (DOT HS-809-012) (http://safety.fhwa.dot.gov/fourthlevel/pdf/809012.pdf, accessed 17 November 2003).

53. *European Road Safety Action Programme. Halving the number of road accident victims in the European Union by 2010: a shared responsibility.* Brussels, Commission of the European Communities, 2003 (Com(2003) 311 final) (http://europa.eu.int/comm/transport/road/roadsafety/rsap/index_en.htm, accessed 17 November 2003).

54. Wang S et al. Trends in road traffic crashes and associated injury and fatality in the People's Republic of China, 1951–1999. *Injury Control and Safety Promotion,* 2003, 10:83–87.

55. Odero W, Khayesi M, Heda PM. Road traffic injuries in Kenya: magnitude, causes and status of intervention. *Injury Control and Safety Promotion,* 2003, 10:53–61.

56. Afukaar FK. Speed control in LMICs: issues, challenges and opportunities in reducing road traffic injuries. *Injury Control and Safety Promotion,* 2003, 10:77–81.

57. *The road to safety 2001–2005: building the foundations of a safe and secure road traffic environment in South Africa.* Pretoria, Ministry of Transport, 2001 (http://www.transport.gov.za/projects/index.html, accessed 17 November 2003).

58. Nafukho FM, Khayesi M. Livelihood, conditions of work, regulation and road safety in the small-scale public transport sector: a case of the *Matatu* mode of transport in Kenya. In: Godard X, Fatonzoun I, eds. *Urban mobility for all. Proceedings of the Tenth International CODATU Conference, Lome, Togo, 12–15 November 2002.* Lisse, AA Balkema Publishers, 2002:241–245.

59. Nantulya VM, Muli-Musiime F. Uncovering the social determinants of road traffic accidents in Kenya. In: Evans T et al., eds. *Challenging inequities: from ethics to action.* Oxford, Oxford University Press, 2001:211–225.

60. Hijar M, Vazquez-Vela E, Arreola-Risa C. Pedestrian traffic injuries in Mexico: a country update. *Injury Control and Safety Promotion,* 2003, 10:37–43.

61. Mohan D. Road safety in less-motorized environments: future concerns. *International Journal of Epidemiology,* 2002, 31:527–532.

62. Crandall JR, Bhalla KS, Madely J. Designing road vehicles for pedestrian protection. *British Medical Journal,* 2002, 324:1145–1148.

63. Allsop RE, ed. *Safety of pedestrians and cyclists in urban areas.* Brussels, European Transport Safety Council, 1999 (http://www.etsc.be/rep.htm, accessed 17 November 2003).

64. *Safety of vulnerable road users.* Paris, Organisation for Economic Co-operation and Development, 2001 (http://www.oecd.org/dataoecd/24/4/2103492.pdf, accessed 17 November 2003).

65. *Police enforcement strategies to reduce traffic casualties in Europe.* Brussels, European Transport Safety Council, 1999.

66. *Promotion of mobility and safety of vulnerable road users. PROMISING.* Leidschendam, Institute for Road Safety Research, 2001.

67. Kandela P. Road accidents in Jordan. *Lancet,* 1993, 342:426.

68. Rodriguez DY, Fernandez FJ, Velasquez HA. Road traffic injuries in Colombia. *Injury Control and Safety Promotion,* 2003, 10:29–35.

69. Hijar M, Trostle J, Bronfman M. Pedestrian injuries in Mexico: a multi-method approach. *Social Science and Medicine,* 2003, 57:2149–2159.

70. Downing A. Pedestrian safety in developing countries. In: *Proceedings of the Vulnerable Road User. International Conference on Traffic Safety, New Delhi, 27–30 January 1991.* New Delhi, Macmillan India, 1991.

71. Mackay GM, Wodzin E. Global priorities for vehicle safety. In: *International Conference on Vehicle Safety 2002: IMechE conference transactions.* London, Institution of Mechanical Engineers, 2002:3–9.

72. Peden M, McGee K, Krug E, eds. *Injury: a leading cause of the global burden of disease, 2000.* Geneva, World Health Organization, 2002 (http://whqlibdoc.who.int/publications/2002/9241562323.pdf, accessed 30 october 2003).

73. Mayhew DR, Simpson HM. *New to the road. Young drivers and novice drivers: similar problems and solutions.* Ottawa, Traffic Injury Research Foundation, 1990.

74. Cerrelli E. *Crash data and rates for age-sex groups of drivers, 1996.* Washington, DC, National Center for Statistics and Analysis, 1998 (NHTSA Research Note).

75. McLean AJ et al. *Regional comparative study of motorcycle accidents with special reference to licensing requirements.* Adelaide, National Health and Medical Research Council Road Accident Research Unit, University of Adelaide, 1990 (Research Report 2/90).

76. Williams AF. Teenage drivers: patterns of risk. *Journal of Safety Research*, 2003, 34:5–15.

77. Lam LT et al. Passenger carriage and car crash injury: a comparison between younger and older drivers. *Accident Analysis and Prevention*, 2003, 35:861–867.

78. Borkenstein RF et al. *The role of the drinking driver in traffic accidents.* Bloomington, IN, Department of Police Administration, Indiana University, 1964.

79. McLean AJ, Holubowycz OT. Alcohol and the risk of accident involvement. In: Goldberg L, ed. *Alcohol, drugs and traffic safety. Proceedings of the 8th International Conference on Alcohol, Drugs and Traffic Safety, Stockholm, 15–19 June 1980.* Stockholm, Almqvist & Wiksell International, 1981: 113–123.

80. Hurst PM, Harte D, Frith WJ. The Grand Rapids dip revisited. *Accident Analysis and Prevention*, 1994, 26:647–654.

81. Moskowitz H, Fiorentino D. *A review of the literature on the effects of low doses of alcohol on driving-related skills.* Washington, DC, National Highway Traffic Safety Administration, 2000 (NHTSA Report No. DOT HS-809-028).

82. Compton RP et al. Crash risk of alcohol impaired driving. In: Mayhew DR, Dussault C, eds. *Proceedings of the 16th International Conference on Alcohol, Drugs and Traffic Safety, Montreal, 4–9 August 2002.* Montreal, Société de l'assurance automobile du Québec, 2002:39–44 (http://www.saaq.gouv.qc.ca/t2002/actes/pdf/(06a).pdf, accessed 17 November 2003).

83. Allsop RE. *Alcohol and road accidents: a discussion of the Grand Rapids study.* Harmondsworth, Road Research Laboratory, 1966 (RRL Report No. 6).

84. Moskowitz H et al. Methodological issues in epidemiological studies of alcohol crash risk. In: Mayhew DR, Dussault C, eds. *Proceedings of the 16th International Conference on Alcohol, Drugs and Traffic Safety, Montreal, 4–9 August 2002.* Montreal, Société de l'assurance automobile du Québec, 2002:45–50 (http://www.saaq.gouv.qc.ca/t2002/actes/pdf/(06a).pdf, accessed 17 November 2003).

85. Haworth NL. Alcohol in motorcycle crashes. In: Laurell H, Schlyter F, eds. *Proceedings of the 15th International Conference on Alcohol, Drugs and Traffic Safety, Stockholm, 22–26 May 2000.* Stockholm, Swedish National Road Administration, 2000 (http://www.vv.se/traf_sak/t2000/316.pdf, accessed 17 November 2003).

86. Zador PL. Alcohol-related relative risk of fatal driver injuries in relation to driver age and sex. *Journal of Studies on Alcohol*, 1991, 52:302–310.

87. Zador PL, Krawchuk SA, Voas RB. *Relative risk of fatal crash involvement by BAC, age, and gender.* Washington, DC, National Highway Traffic Safety Administration, 2000 (DOT HS-809-050).

88. Keall MD, Frith WJ, Patterson TL. The influence of alcohol, age and number of passengers on the night-time risk of driver fatal injury in New Zealand. *Accident Analysis and Prevention*, 2004, 36:49–61.

89. Maycock G. *Drinking and driving in Great Britain: a review.* Crowthorne, Transport Research Laboratory, 1997 (TRL Report 232).

90. Stewart K et al. International comparisons of laws and alcohol crash rates: lessons learned. In: *Proceedings of the 15th International Conference on Alcohol, Drugs and Traffic Safety, Stockholm, 22–26 May 2000.* Stockholm, Swedish National Road Administration, 2000 (http://www.vv.se/traf_sak/t2000/541.pdf, accessed on 17 November 2003).

91. *Reducing traffic injuries resulting from alcohol impairment.* Brussels, European Transport Safety Council, Working Party on Road User Behaviour, 1995.

92. Gledec M. The presence of alcohol in Croatian road traffic. In: *Proceedings of the 15th International Conference on Alcohol, Drugs and Traffic Safety, Stockholm, 22–26 May 2000.* Stockholm, Swedish National Road Administration, 2000 (http://www.vv.se/traf_sak/t2000/314.pdf, accessed 17 November 2003).

93. Mock CN, Asiamah G, Amegashie J. A random, roadside breathalyzer survey of alcohol impaired drivers in Ghana. *Journal of Crash Prevention and Injury Control*, 2001, 2:193–202.

94. Mishra BK, Banerji AK, Mohan D. Two-wheeler injuries in Delhi, India: a study of crash victims hospitalized in a neuro-surgery ward. *Accident Analysis and Prevention*, 1984, 16:407–416.

95. Mathijssen MPM. *Rijden onder invloed in Nederland, 1996–1997: ontwikkeling van het alcoholgebruik door automobilisten in weekendnachten [Driving under the influence in the Netherlands, 1996–1997: changes in car driver alcohol use during weekend nights]*. Leidschendam, Institute for Road Safety Research, 1998 (SWOV Report R-98-37).

96. Davis A et al. *Improving road safety by reducing impaired driving in LMICs: a scoping study*. Crowthorne, Transport Research Laboratory, 2003 (Project Report 724/03).

97. Odero WO, Zwi AB. Alcohol-related traffic injuries and fatalities in LMICs: a critical review of literature. In: Kloeden CN, McLean AJ, eds. *Proceedings of the 13th International Conference on Alcohol, Drugs and Traffic Safety, Adelaide, 13–18 August 1995*. Adelaide, Road Accident Research Unit, 1995:713–720.

98. Peden M et al. Injured pedestrians in Cape Town: the role of alcohol. *South African Medical Journal*, 1996, 16:1103–1105.

99. Peden M et al. Substance abuse and trauma in Cape Town. *South African Medical Journal*, 2000, 90:251–255.

100. *Traffic safety facts, 2000: Motorcycles*. Washington, DC, National Highway Traffic Safety Administration, 2001 (DOT HS-809-326).

101. Koornstra M et al. *Sunflower: a comparative study of the development of road safety in Sweden, the United Kingdom and the Netherlands*. Leidschendam, Institute for Road Safety Research, 2002.

102. Ross HL. *Deterring the drinking driver: legal policy and social control*. Lexington, DC Heath, 1984.

103. Suriyawongpaisal P, Plitapolkarnpim A, Tawonwanchai A. Application of 0.05 per cent legal blood alcohol limits to traffic injury control in Bangkok. *Journal of the Medical Association of Thailand*, 2002, 85:496–501.

104. Clayton AB, Colgan MA, Tunbridge RJ. The role of the drinking pedestrian in traffic accidents. In: *Proceedings of 15th International Conference on Alcohol, Drugs and Traffic Safety, Stockholm, 22–26 May 2000*. Stockholm, Swedish National Road Administration, 2000 (http://www.vv.se/traf_sak/t2000/553.pdf, accessed on 7 December 2003).

105. Holubowycz OT. Alcohol-involved pedestrians: the Australian experience. In: Kloeden CN, McLean AJ, eds. *Proceedings of the 13th International Conference on Alcohol, Drugs and Traffic Safety, Adelaide, 13–18 August 1995*. Adelaide, Road Accident Research Unit, 1995:700–710.

106. Keigan M et al. *The incidence of alcohol in fatally injured adult pedestrians*. Crowthorne, Transport Research Laboratory, 2003 (TRL Report 579).

107. Everest JT. *The involvement of alcohol in fatal accidents to adult pedestrians*. Crowthorne, Transport Research Laboratory, 1992 (RR 343).

108. Hunter CE et al. *The prevalence and role of alcohol, cannabinoids, benzodiazepines and stimulants in non-fatal crashes*. Adelaide, Forensic Science, Department for Administrative and Information Services, 1998.

109. Moskowitz H. Marijuana and driving. *Accident Analysis and Prevention*, 1985, 17:323–346.

110. Ellinwood EHJR, Heatherly DG. Benzodiazepines, the popular minor tranquilizers: dynamics of effect on driving skills. *Accident Analysis and Prevention*, 1985, 17:283–290.

111. Judd LL. The effect of antipsychotic drugs on driving and driving-related psychomotor functions. *Accident Analysis and Prevention*, 1985, 17:319–322.

112. Hemmelgarn B et al. Benzodiazepine use and the risk of motor vehicle crash in the elderly. *Journal of the American Medical Association*, 1997, 277: 27–31.

113. McKenna FP. The human factor in driving accidents: an overview of approaches and problems. *Ergonomics*, 1982, 25:867–877.

114. Mørland J et al. Driving under the influence of drugs: an increasing problem. In: Kloeden CN, McLean AJ, eds. *Proceedings of the 13th International Conference on Alcohol, Drugs and Traffic Safety, Adelaide, 13–18 August 1995*. Adelaide, Road Accident Research Unit, 1995:780–784.

115. Christophersen AS et al. Recidivism among drugged drivers in Norway. In: Mercier-Guyon C, ed. *Proceedings of the 14th International Conference on Alcohol, Drugs and Traffic Safety, Annecy, France, 21–26 September 1997.* Annecy, Centre d'études et de recherches en médecine du trafic, 1997:803–807.

116. Moskowitz H. Marijuana and driving. *Accident Analysis and Prevention*, 1976, 8:21–26.

117. Robbe JHW. *Influence of marijuana on driving.* [unpublished thesis]. Limburg, University of Limburg, 1994.

118. Mura P et al. Comparison of the prevalence of alcohol, cannabis and other drugs between 900 injured drivers and 900 control subjects: results of a French collaborative study. *Forensic Science International,* 2003, 133:79–85.

119. Sexton BF et al. *The influence of cannabis and alcohol on driving.* Crowthorne, Transport Research Laboratory, 2002 (TRL Report 543) (http://www.trl.co.uk/abstracts/543summary.pdf, accessed 17 November 2003).

120. Hartley LR, Arnold PK. *Recommendations from the Second International Conference on Fatigue in Transportation, Fremantle, Western Australia, 11–16 February 1996.* Fremantle, Institute for Safety and Transport, Murdoch University, Western Australia, 1996 (Report 113).

121. National Center on Sleep Disorders Research/ National Highway Traffic Safety Administration Expert Panel on Driver Fatigue and Sleepiness. *Drowsy driving and automobile crashes.* Washington, DC, National Highway Traffic Safety Administration, 1996 (http://www.nhtsa.dot.gov/people/injury/drowsy_driving1/Drowsy.html, accessed 17 November 2003).

122. Connor J et al. Driver sleepiness and risk of serious injury to car occupants: population-based control study. *British Medical Journal*, 2002, 324:1125.

123. Mock C, Amegashi J, Darteh K. Role of commercial drivers in motor vehicle related injuries in Ghana. *Injury Prevention,* 1999, 5:268–271.

124. *Fatigue, alcohol, other drugs, and medical factors in fatal-to-the-driver heavy truck crashes. Volume 1.* Washington, DC, National Transportation Safety Board, 1990 (Safety Report NTSB SS–90/01).

125. *Factors that affect fatigue in heavy truck accidents.* Washington, DC, National Transportation Safety Board, 1995 (Safety Report NTSB SS–95/01).

126. *Evaluation of U.S. Department of Transportation efforts in the 1990s to address operator fatigue.* Washington, DC, National Transportation Safety Board, 1999 (Safety report NTSB/SR–99/01) (http://www.ntsb.gov/publictn/1999/SR9901.pdf, accessed 17 November 2003).

127. McDonald N, ed. *The role of driver fatigue in commercial road transport crashes.* Brussels, European Transport Safety Council, 2001.

128. Hamelin P. Lorry drivers' time habits in work and their involvement in traffic accidents. *Ergonomics*, 1987, 30:1323–1333.

129. *The risk of using a mobile phone while driving.* Birmingham, Royal Society for the Prevention of Accidents, 2002.

130. Zwahlen HT, Adams CC, Schwartz PJ. Safety aspects of cellular telephones in automobiles. In: *Proceedings of the 18th International Symposium on Automotive Technology and Automation, Vol. 1, Florence.* Croydon, Allied Automation, 1988.

131. Brown ID, Tickner AH, Simmonds DCV. Interference between concurrent tasks of driving and telephoning. *Journal of Applied Psychology,* 1969, 53:419–424.

132. Alm H, Nilsson L. The effect of a mobile telephone task on driver behaviour in a car following situation. *Accident Analysis and Prevention*, 1995, 27:707–715.

133. Alm H, Nilsson L. Changes in driver behaviour as a function of handsfree mobile phones: a simulator study. *Accident Analysis and Prevention*, 1994, 26:441–451.

134. *An investigation of the safety implications of wireless communication in vehicles.* Washington, DC, National Highway Traffic Safety Administration, 1997 (http://www.nhtsa.dot.gov/people/injury/research/wireless/, accessed 17 November 2003).

135. Redelmeier DA, Tibshirani RJ. Association between cellular-telephone calls and motor vehicle collisions. *New England Journal of Medicine,* 1997, 336:453–458.

136. Koornstra MJ. Safety relevance of vision research and theory. In: Gale AG et al., eds. *Vision in vehicles IV.* Amsterdam, Elsevier, 1993:3–13.

137. Henderson RL et al. *Motor vehicle conspicuity.* Detroit, MI, Society of Automotive Engineers, 1983 (Society of Automotive Engineers Technical Paper Series 830566).

138. Williams MJ, Hoffman ER. Motorcycle conspicuity and traffic accidents. *Accident Analysis and Prevention,* 1979, 11:209–211.

139. Elvik R. A meta-analysis of studies concerning the safety effects of daytime running lights on cars. *Accident Analysis and Prevention,* 1996, 28:685–694.

140. Gwehenberger J et al. Injury risk for truck occupants due to serious commercial vehicle accidents – results of real-world-crash analysis. In: *Proceedings of 2002 International IRCOBI Conference on Biomechanics of Impact, Munich, 18–20 September 2002.* Bron, Institut National de Recherche sur les Transports et leur Sécurité, 2002:105–118.

141. Chawla A et al. Safer truck front design for pedestrian impacts. *Journal of Crash Prevention and Injury Control,* 2000, 2:33–43.

142. Hurt HH, Quellet JV, Thomas DR. *Motorcycle accident cause factors and the identification of countermeasures.* Washington, DC, National Highway Traffic Safety Administration, 1981 (DOT HS 805-862-3).

143. Radin Umar RS, Mackay GM, Hills BL. Preliminary analysis of motorcycle accidents: short-term impacts of the running headlights campaign and regulation in Malaysia. *Journal of Traffic Medicine,* 1995, 23:17–28.

144. Radin Umar RS, Mackay GM, Hills BL. Modelling of conspicuity-related motorcycle accidents in Seremban and Shah Alam, Malaysia. *Accident Analysis and Prevention,* 1996, 28:325–332.

145. Schoon CC. *Invloed kwaliteit fiets op ongevallen [The influence of cycle quality in crashes].* Leidschendam, Institute for Road Safety Research, 1996 (SWOV Report R-96-32).

146. Roberts I, Power C. Does the decline in child injury death rates vary by class? *British Medical Journal,* 1996, 313:784–786.

147. *Low cost road and traffic engineering measures for casualty reduction.* Brussels, European Transport Safety Council, 1996.

148. Ross A et al., eds. *Towards safer roads in developing countries: A guide for planners and engineers.* Crowthorne, Transport Research Laboratory, 1991.

149. Khayesi M. *An analysis of the pattern of road traffic accidents in relation to selected socio-economic dynamics and intervention measures in Kenya* [unpublished thesis]. Nairobi, Kenyatta University, 1999.

150. Kanianthra JN. Advanced technologies: the pathway to total safety. In: *18th Enhanced Safety of Vehicles Technical Conference, Nagoya, Japan, 19 May 2003.* Washington, DC, National Highway Traffic Safety Administration, 2003 (http://www-nrd.nhtsa.dot.gov/departments/nrd-01/esv/18th/discussions/JK_ESVAdv.html, accessed 2 December 2003).

151. Van Schoor O, van Niekerk J, Grobbelaar B. Mechanical failures as a contributing cause to motor vehicle accidents: South Africa. *Accident Analysis and Prevention,* 2001, 33:713–721.

152. O'Neill B et al. The World Bank's global road safety and partnership. *Traffic Injury Prevention,* 2002, 3:190–194.

153. Jones IS, Stein HS. Defective equipment and tractor-trailer crash involvement. *Accident Analysis and Prevention,* 1989, 21:469–481.

154. Hobbs CA, ed. *Priorities for EU motor vehicle safety design.* Brussels, European Transport Safety Council, Working Party on Vehicle Safety Priorities for EU Motor Vehicle Safety Design, 2001.

155. *Collision and consequence.* Stockholm, Swedish National Roads Administration, 2003.

156. Blows S et al. Vehicle year and the risk of car crash injury. *Injury Prevention,* 2003, 9:353–356.

157. Brainard B. Injury profiles in pedestrian motor vehicle trauma. *Annals of Emergency Medicine,* 1986, 18:881–883.

158. Kajzer J, Yang JK, Mohan D. Safer bus fronts for pedestrian impact protection in bus-pedestrian accidents. In: *Proceedings of the International Research Council on Biomechanics of Impact (IRCOBI) Conference, Verona, Italy, 9–11 September 1992.* Bron, International Research Council on the Biomechanics of Impact, 1992:13–23.

159. Mackay M. Engineering in accidents: vehicle design and injuries. *Injury,* 1994, 25:615–621.

160. *Improved test methods to evaluate pedestrian protection afforded by passenger cars.* European Enhanced Vehicle-safety Committee, EEVC Working Group 17, 1998 (http://www.eevc.org/publicdocs/WG17_Improved_test_methods_updated_

sept_2002.pdf, accessed 1 December 2002).

161. European New Car Assessment Programme (Euro-NCAP) [web site]. (http://www.euroncap.com/results.htm, accessed on 17 November 2003).

162. Australian New Car Assessment Programme [web site]. (http://www.mynrma.com.au/motoring/cars/crash_tests/ancap/, accessed 17 November 2003).

163. Mackay M. Leg injuries to MTW riders and motorcycle design. In: *20th Annual Proceedings of the American Association for Automotive Medicine, Washington, DC, 7–9 October 1985.* Washington, DC, American Association for Automotive Medicine, 1985:169–180.

164. Pang TY, Radin Umar RS, Azhar A. Relative risk of fatal injury in the high-performance small motorcycles (HPSM) in Malaysia. *Journal of Crash Prevention and Injury Control*, 2001, 2:307–315.

165. *Report on motorcycle safety.* Brussels, European Experimental Vehicles Committee, 1993.

166. Barss P et al. *Injury prevention: an international perspective, epidemiology, surveillance and policy.* Oxford, Oxford University Press, 1998.

167. Joach AW. *Vehicle design and compatibility.* Washington, DC, National Highway Traffic Safety Administration, 2000 (DOT HS-809-194).

168. O'Neill B, Mohan D. Reducing motor vehicle crash deaths and injuries in newly motorising countries. *British Medical Journal*, 2002, 324:1142–1145.

169. Servadei F et al. Effect of Italy's motorcycle helmet law on traumatic brain injuries. *Injury Prevention*, 2003, 9:257–260.

170. *Motorcycle safety helmets. COST 327.* Brussels, Commission of the European Communities, 2001 (http://www.cordis.lu/cost-transport/src/cost-327.htm, accessed 17 November 2003).

171. Radin Umar RS. Helmet initiatives in Malaysia. In: *Proceedings of the 2nd World Engineering Congress.* Sarawak, Institution of Engineers, 2002:93–101.

172. Kulanthayan S et al. Compliance of proper safety helmet usage in motorcyclists. *Medical Journal of Malaysia,* 2000, 55:40–44.

173. Ichikawa M, Chadbunchachai W, Marui E. Effect of the helmet act for MTW riders in Thailand. *Accident Analysis and Prevention*, 2003, 35:183–189.

174. Mohan D. A study of helmet and motorised two-wheeler use patterns in Delhi. *Indian Highways*, 1983, 11:8–16.

175. Glassbrenner D. *Safety belt and helmet use in 2002: overall results.* Washington, DC, National Highway Traffic Safety Administration, 2002 (DOT HS-809-500).

176. Conrad P et al. Helmets, injuries and cultural definitions: motorcycle injury in urban Indonesia. *Accident Analysis and Prevention*, 1996, 28:193–200.

177. Ong WY. *Design of motorcycle crash helmet for children.* [unpublished thesis]. Serdang, Universiti Putra Malaysia, 2001.

178. Peek-Asa C, McArthur DL, Kraus JF. The prevalence of non-standard helmet use and head injuries among motorcycle riders. *Accident Analysis and Prevention*, 1999, 31:229–233.

179. Nixon J et al. Bicycle accidents in childhood. *British Medical Journal*, 1987, 294:1267–1269.

180. Thomas S et al. Effectiveness of bicycle helmets in preventing head injury in children: case-control study. *British Medical Journal*, 1994, 308:173–176.

181. Thompson DC, Rivara FP, Thompson RS. Effectiveness of bicycle safety helmets in preventing head injuries: a case-control study. *Journal of the American Medical Association*, 1996, 276:1968–1973.

182. Sosin DM, Sacks JJ, Webb KW. Pediatric head injuries and deaths from bicycling in the United States. *Pediatrics*, 1996, 98:868–870.

183. Attewell RG, Glase K, McFadden M. Bicycle helmet efficacy: a meta-analysis. *Accident Analysis and Prevention*, 2001, 33:345–352.

184. Weiss BD. Cycle related head injuries. *Clinics in Sport Medicine*, 1994, 13:99–112.

185. Mackay M. The use of seat belts: some behavioural considerations. *Proceedings of the risk-taking behaviour and traffic safety symposium, 19–22 October 1997.* Washington, DC, National Highway Traffic Safety Administration, 1997:1–14.

186. *Seat-belts and child restraints: increasing use and optimising performance.* Brussels, European Transport Safety Council, 1996.

187. Cummings P et al. Association of driver air bags with driver fatality: a matched cohort study. *British Medical Journal*, 2002, 324:119–122.

188. Evans L. Restraint effectiveness, occupant ejection from cars and fatality reductions. *Accident Analysis and Prevention*, 1990, 22:167–175.

189. Valtonen J. *The use of safety belts and their effect in accidents.* Helsinki, Central Organization for Traffic Safety, 1991.

190. Kamrèn B. *Seat belt use among fatally injured in the county of Stockholm 1991–1992.* Stockholm, Folksam, 1992.

191. Hill JR, Mackay GM, Morris AP. Chest and abdominal injuries caused by seat belt loading. In: *Proceedings of the 36th Annual Conference of the Association for the Advancement of Automotive Medicine (AAAM), Portland, October 1992.* Chicago, Association for Advancement of Automotive Medicine, 1992: 25–41.

192. *Behavioural adaptations to changes in the road transport system.* Paris, Organisation for Economic Co-operation and Development, 1990.

193. Huguenin RD. Does the use of seat belts lead to "compensatory" behaviour? In: *Proceedings of the 26th International Symposium on Automotive Technology and Automation, Aachen, Germany, 13–17 September 1993.* Croydon, Automotive Automation Ltd, 1993:365–372.

194. Mäkinen T, Wittink RD, Hagenzieker MP. *The use of seat belts and contributing factors: an international comparison.* Leidschendam, Institute for Road Safety Research, 1991 (SWOV Report R-91-30).

195. Yang B, Kim J. Road traffic accidents and policy interventions in Korea. *Injury Control and Safety Promotion*, 2003, 10:89–94.

196. Silveira AJ. Seat belt use in Argentina: a 10-year struggle. *Traffic Injury Prevention*, 2003, 4:173–175.

197. Van Kampen LTB. Seat belt research and legislation in the Netherlands. In: *Proceedings of the 10th International Technical Conference on Experimental Safety Vehicles, Oxford, 1–4 July 1985.* Washington, DC, National Highway Traffic Safety Administration, 1985:560–567.

198. *Traffic safety facts 2002: children.* Washington, DC, National Highway Traffic Safety Administration, 2002 (DOT HS-809-607).

199. Malm S et al. Hurkan vi skydda barn i bil? [How to protect children in cars?] In: *Trafiksäkerhet ur ett Nollvisionsperspektiv seminar,* Stockholm, Folksam, 2001.

200. Crandall CS, Olson LM, Sklar DP. Mortality reduction with air bag and seat belt use in head-on passenger car collisions. *American Journal of Epidemiology*, 2001, 153:219–224.

201. Ferguson SA, Lund AK, Greene MA. *Driver fatalities in 1985–94 airbag cars.* Arlington, VA, Insurance Institute for Highway Safety, 1995.

202. *Fifth/sixth report to Congress: effectiveness of occupant protection systems and their use.* Washington, DC, National Highway Traffic Safety Administration, 2001 (DOT HS-809-442)(http://www.nrd.nhtsa.dot.go/pdf/nrd-30/NSCA/Rpts/2002/809-442.pdf, accessed 10 December 2003).

203. Aldman B, Andersson A, Saxmark O. Possible effects of airbag inflation on a standing child. In: *Proceedings of 18th American Association for Automotive Medicine (AAAM) Conference, Toronto, Canada, 12–14 September 1974.* Washington, DC, American Association for Automotive Medicine, 1974:15–29.

204. Anund A et al. *Child safety in care – literature review.* Linköping, Sweden, Swedish National Road and Transport Research Institute, 2003 (VTI report 489A9 (http://www.vti.se/PDF/reports/R489A.pdf, accessed on 7 December 2003).

205. Weber K. Rear-facing restraint for small child passengers. *University of Michigan Transportation Research Institute Research Reviews*, 1995, 25:12–17.

206. Schoon CC, Huijskens CG, Heijkamp AH. Misuse of restraint systems for children in the Netherlands. In: *Proceedings of the 1992 International Conference on the Biomechanics of Impacts (IRCOBI), Verona, Italy, 9–11 September 1992.* Bron, International Research Council on the Biomechanics of Impact, 1992:385–393.

207. Koch D, Medgyesi M, Landry P. *Saskatchewan's occupant restraint program (1988–94): performance to date.* Regina, Saskatchewan Government Insurance, 1995.

208. Kloeden CN et al. *Severe and fatal car crashes due to roadside hazards: a report to the motor accident commission.* Adelaide, University of Adelaide, National Health and Medical Research Council, Road Accident Research Unit, 1998.

209. *Forgiving roadsides*. Brussels, European Transport Safety Council, 1998.

210. Mock CN, nii-Amon-Kotei D, Maier RV. Low utilization of formal medical services by injured persons in a developing nation: health service data underestimate the importance of trauma. *Journal of Trauma*, 1997, 42:504–513.

211. Hussain IM, Redmond AD. Are pre-hospital deaths from accidental injury preventable? *British Medical Journal*, 1994, 308:1077–1080.

212. Buylaert W, ed. *Reducing injuries from post-impact care*. Brussels, European Transport Safety Council, Working Party on Post Impact Care, 1999.

213. Mock CN et al. Trauma mortality patterns in three nations at different economic levels: implications for global trauma system development. *Journal of Trauma*, 1998, 44:804–814.

214. McKibbin B et al. *The management of skeletal trauma in the United Kingdom*. London, British Orthopaedic Association, 1992.

215. Forjuoh S et al. Transport of the injured to hospitals in Ghana: the need to strengthen the practice of trauma care. *Pre-hospital Immediate Care*, 1999, 3:66–70.

216. Nantulya VM, Reich MR. The neglected epidemic: road traffic injuries in developing countries. *British Medical Journal*, 2002, 324:1139–1141.

217. Becker LR et al. Relative risk of injury and death in ambulances and other emergency vehicles. *Accident Analysis and Prevention*, 2003, 35:941–948.

218. Arreola-Risa C, Speare JOR. Trauma in Mexico. *Trauma Quarterly*, 1999, 14:211–220.

219. MacGowan WA. Surgical manpower worldwide. *Bulletin of the American College of Surgeons*, 1987, 72:5–9.

CHAPTER 4

Interventions

A road traffic system designed for safe, sustainable use

Road traffic deaths and serious injuries are to a great extent preventable, since the risk of incurring injury in a crash is largely predictable and many countermeasures, proven to be effective, exist. Road traffic injury needs to be considered alongside heart disease, cancer and stroke as a preventable public health problem that responds well to targeted interventions (*1*).

The provision of safe, sustainable and affordable means of travel is a key objective in the planning and design of road traffic systems. To achieve it requires firm political will, and an integrated approach involving close collaboration of many sectors, in which the health sector plays a full and active role. In such a systems-based approach, it is possible at the same time to tackle other major problems associated with road traffic, such as congestion, noise emission, air pollution and lack of physical exercise (*2*).

Progress is being made in many parts of the world where multisectoral strategic plans are leading to incremental reductions in the number of road deaths and injuries (*3, 4*). Such strategies address the three prime elements of the traffic system – vehicles, road users and the road infrastructure. Vehicle and road engineering measures need to take into account the safety needs and physical limitations of road users. Vehicle technology needs to consider roadside equipment. Measures involving the road infrastructure must be compatible with the characteristics of vehicles. Vehicle measures should be complemented by appropriate behaviour on the part of road users, such as wearing seat-belts. In all these strategies, managing speed is a fundamental factor.

This chapter provides an overview of the wide range of interventions for road safety, examining what is known about their practicability, effectiveness, cost and acceptability to the public. Proven interventions in one setting, of course, may not easily be transferable elsewhere, but will instead require careful adaptation and evaluation. Where effective interventions are altogether lacking, scientific research is needed to develop and test new measures.

Managing exposure to risk through transport and land-use policies

Perhaps the least used of all road safety intervention strategies are those that aim to reduce exposure to risk. Yet the underlying factors determining exposure to risk can have important effects (*5*). While further research is required to fully explore intervention strategies, it is known that exposure to road injury risk can be decreased by strategies that include:

— reducing the volume of motor vehicle traffic by means of better land use;
— providing efficient networks where the shortest or quickest routes coincide with the safest routes;
— encouraging people to switch from higher-risk to lower-risk modes of transport;
— placing restrictions on motor vehicle users, on vehicles, or on the road infrastructure.

The impact of strategies aimed at influencing mobility and access tends to be cumulative and mutually reinforcing, and such strategies can most effectively be implemented in combination. In high-income countries, it has been estimated that a comprehensive programme with a complementary set of cost-effective measures could reduce the total amount of car travel, per capita, by 20–40% (*6*). Many countries are now addressing these issues, mainly in the interests of sustainable mobility. Bogotá in Colombia, for instance, has attempted to reduce exposure to risk through measures that include a mass transit programme for vulnerable road users and restrictions on motor vehicle access to the city during certain times (*7, 8*).

Reducing motor vehicle traffic
Efficient land use

The organization of land use affects the number of trips people make, by what means they choose to travel, the length of trips and the route taken (*9*). Different land use creates different sets of traffic patterns (*10*). The main aspects of land use that influence road safety are (*9*):

— the spatial distribution of origins and destinations of road journeys;

— urban population density and patterns of urban growth;
— the configuration of the road network;
— the size of residential areas;
— alternatives to private motorized transport.

Land-use planning practices and "smart growth" land-use policies – development of high-density, compact buildings with easily accessible services and amenities – can serve to lessen the exposure risk of road users. The creation of clustered, mixed-use community services, for example, can cut the distances between commonly used destinations, curtailing the need to travel and reducing dependence on private motor vehicles (6).

Safety impact assessments of transport and land-use plans

Evaluations of the impact on safety of transport projects usually focus on the individual project, with little consideration of the effect on the wider network (11). This can result in strategies for improving mobility, reducing congestion and improving the environment that are incompatible with road safety. The likely effects of planning decisions to do with transport or land use on the *whole* of the road network should therefore be considered at an early stage, to avoid unintended, adverse consequences for road safety (9, 10, 12).

Area-wide safety impact assessments should be routinely conducted at the same time as other assessments of policies and projects related to transport and land use. Safety impact assessments are not yet carried out either routinely or systematically in most places, though there has been experience with them in the Netherlands, and to some extent elsewhere (13).

Providing shorter, safer routes

In an efficient road network, exposure to crash risk can be minimized by ensuring that trips are short and routes direct, and that the quickest routes are also the safest routes. Route management techniques can achieve these objectives by decreasing travel times on desired routes, increasing travel times on undesired routes, and re-directing traf-

fic (14). Having to take a detour in a car means that extra fuel will be used, but for pedestrians it means extra physical exertion. There is thus a strong incentive to find the easiest and most direct route. Studies have, in fact, shown that pedestrians and cyclists place a higher value on journey time than do drivers or those using public transport – a finding that should be reflected in planning decisions (15, 16).

Safe crossing facilities for pedestrians and cyclists are likely not to be used if many steps need to be climbed, if long detours are involved, or if the crossings are poorly lit or underpasses badly maintained. A study in Brazil showed that many pedestrians who had been struck by vehicles had chosen to climb over central traffic-lane barriers, rather than climb a flight of stairs to a footbridge (17). Interviews with pedestrian crash survivors in Mexico found that one of the main underlying risk factors was the presence of bridges that were poorly located or regarded as unsafe (18). In Uganda, the construction of an overpass for pedestrians on a major highway in Kampala had little effect either on pedestrian road behaviour or on the incidence of crashes and injuries because of its inappropriate location (19).

Trip reduction measures

It has been estimated from studies in high-income countries that, under certain conditions, for each 1% reduction in motor vehicle distance travelled, there is a corresponding 1.4–1.8% reduction in the incidence of crashes (20, 21). Measures that may reduce the distance travelled include:
— making greater use of electronic means of communications as a substitute for delivering communications by road;
— encouraging more people to work from home, using e-mail to communicate with their workplace;
— better management of commuter transport, and of transport to and from schools and colleges;
— better management of tourist transport;
— bans on freight transport;
— restrictions on vehicle parking and road use.

Encouraging use of safer modes of travel

Whether measured by the time spent travelling or by the number of trips, travel by bus and train is many times safer than any other mode of road travel. Policies that stimulate the use of public transport, and its combination with walking and cycling, are thus to be encouraged. While the walking and cycling parts of journeys bear relatively high risks, pedestrians and cyclists create less risk for other road users than do motor vehicles (*6*). However, by implementing known safety measures, it should be possible to achieve a growth in healthier forms of travel, such as walking and cycling, and at the same time reduce the incidence of deaths and injuries among pedestrians and cyclists. These are goals that are increasingly being adopted in national transport policies in high-income countries (*15*).

Strategies that may increase the use of public transport include (*6*):

— improved mass transit systems (including improvements to routes covered and ticketing procedures, shorter distances between stops, and greater comfort and safety of both the vehicle and the waiting areas);
— better coordination between different modes of travel (including the coordination of schedules and the harmonization of tariff schemes);
— secure shelters for bicycles;
— allowing bicycles to be carried on board trains, ferries and buses;
— "park and ride" facilities, where users can park their cars near public transport stops;
— improvements to taxi services;
— higher fuel taxes and other pricing reforms that discourage private car use in favour of public transport.

Financial incentives have proved successful in some highly-motorized countries; for example, in the Netherlands, a free public transport pass for students has resulted in lower car use (*22*).

In many low-income countries, however, public transport services often operate without regulation and create unacceptable levels of risk, both for their occupants and for those outside the vehicle. These risks arise from overloaded vehicles, long working hours of drivers, speeding and other dangerous behaviour. All

the same, an improved public transport system with proper regulation and enforcement, combined with non-motorized transportation – cycling and walking – can play an important part in low-income and middle-income countries as a response to the growing demand for transport and accessibility.

Despite the generally lower injury risks associated with public transport, more research on the effectiveness of public transport strategies in reducing the incidence of road traffic injuries still needs to be carried out.

Minimizing exposure to high-risk scenarios

Restricting access to different parts of the road network

Preventing pedestrians and cyclists from accessing motorways and preventing motor vehicles from entering pedestrian zones are two well-established measures for minimizing contact between high-speed traffic and unprotected road users. Because vehicles are physically prevented from entering them, pedestrian zones are safer for travel on foot and also – where there is shared use – for bicycle travel. Motorways have the lowest crash rates, in terms of distance travelled, of the whole road network, by virtue of their sole use by motor vehicles, and their use of clear separation of traffic and segregated junctions.

Giving priority in the road network to higher occupancy vehicles

Giving vehicles with many occupants priority in traffic over those with few occupants is a means of reducing the overall distance travelled by private motorized transport – and hence of cutting down on exposure to risk. This strategy is adopted by many cities worldwide. For example, the high-capacity bus system in the city of Curitibá, Brazil, provides segregated bus lanes, priority at traffic lights for buses, as well as safe and fast access for users (*23*).

Restrictions on speed and engine performance of motorized two-wheelers

Many high-income countries have introduced regulations relating to speed and engine performance for mopeds and motorcycles, with the aim of reducing rates of crashes and injury (*24*).

Restricting the engine capacity for beginner motorcyclists has proved to be a successful intervention. In the United Kingdom in the early 1980s, for instance, the maximum engine size of a motorcycle that learners could ride was reduced from 250 cc to 125 cc; this was accompanied by a limitation on the maximum power output (to 9 kW). As a result, many inexperienced motorcyclists transferred to less powerful vehicles, leading to an estimated 25% reduction in casualties among young motorcyclists (*25*). A later study found a significantly greater crash risk associated with larger motorcycles, despite the fact that these machines were ridden mostly by more experienced riders (*25*).

Japan is one country that imposes limits, for safety reasons, on the engine size and performance of large motorcycles used domestically, though similar controls do not apply to exports of new motorcycles from Japan to other countries (*26*). In the case of these exported motorcycles, outputs of 75–90 brake horse power (56–67 kW) – or even 130 brake horse power (97 kW) – are quite common now, with top speeds reaching almost 200 miles/h (322 km/h) (*27*).

Increasing the legal age for use of motorized two-wheelers

In Malaysia, out of a number of proposed measures to reduce motorcycle crashes, increasing the legal riding age from 16 to 18 years was found to have the greatest cost–benefit. Preventing young riders from riding at night was also considered. Although this measure also produced a positive net benefit, the magnitude of the saving was small, since most crashes occurred during daytime (*28*).

Graduated driver licensing systems

The high risks faced by young drivers and motorized two-wheeler riders in their first months of driving have already been discussed (see Chapter 3). For young car drivers, the two principal risks are night-time driving and transporting young passengers (*29*). In response, graduated driver licensing systems were first introduced in New Zealand in 1987, and are now widely implemented in Canada, the United States and some other places. These schemes provide gradual access to a full driving licence for novice drivers and riders (*30*) (see Box 4.1).

BOX 4.1

Graduated driver licensing systems

Beginner drivers of all ages lack both driving skills and experience in recognizing potential dangers. For newly-licensed teenage drivers, their immaturity and limited driving experience result in disproportionately high rates of crashes. Graduated driver licensing systems address the high risks faced by new drivers by requiring an apprenticeship of planned and supervised practice – the learner's permit stage. This is then followed by a provisional licence that places temporary restrictions on unsupervised driving (*31*). Commonly imposed restrictions include limits on night-time driving, limits on the number of passengers, and a prohibition against driving after drinking any alcohol. These restrictions are lifted as new drivers gain experience and teenage drivers mature, gaining a full licence (*32*). Although the specific requirements for advancing through these three stages – the learner's permit, the provisional licence and the full licence – vary according to country, they provide a protective environment while new drivers become more experienced (*33*).

Graduated driver licensing schemes have consistently proved effective in reducing crash risks for new drivers. Peer-reviewed evaluations of the effectiveness of such schemes in Canada, New Zealand and the United States have reported reductions in crashes involving new drivers in the range of 9–43% (*34–36*). Why such reductions should exist has not yet been definitively established. It is generally accepted, though, that the safety benefits of schemes result both from decreases in the amount of driving by inexperienced drivers and from improvements in their driving skills under conditions of low risk.

The elevated risk of a crash for beginner drivers is universal, and graduated driver licensing can effectively reduce this risk. It can apply to all newly-licensed drivers, not just those who are young. Research has clearly demonstrated that older beginner drivers experience higher crash rates than drivers of the same age with several years of experience. For this reason, Canada, where many new drivers are not young, applies graduated driver licensing to all beginners, regardless of their age. Even countries where the legal age for driving is higher than the average can benefit from the introduction of graduated driver licensing.

The reduction in the incidence of crashes resulting from the introduction of these systems varies from 4% to over 60%. This large range may in part be explained by methodological differences, differences in the restrictions used and the degree to which they are enforced (*35*). The major reductions would seem to arise from more supervised driving and from a high degree of compliance with restrictions (*37*). It is not as yet clear, though, which of the many restrictions – including limits on the number of passengers carried, use of seat-belts, lower blood alcohol concentration (BAC) limits and night-time driving bans – is the most cost-effective (*35*). Graduated driver licensing schemes have generally been well accepted (*29*).

The New Zealand scheme is made up of three stages, and all new drivers aged 15–24 years have to take part. The first stage is a six-month supervised learner driver permit, which is obtained by passing a written test, an oral theory test and an eyesight test. The restricted licence stage lasts for 18 months and is completed by passing a practical driving test. There are bans during both the first two stages on night-time driving (from 22:00 to 05:00) and on carrying passengers under the age of 20 years (unless the driving is supervised), as well as a BAC limit of 0.03 g/dl. Violations of these conditions can result in the licence restrictions being extended by a further six months. An evaluation of the scheme found that it had led to an 8% reduction in crashes involving serious injury, and that the restrictions, particularly the night-time driving ban, had made a significant contribution (*36*).

Another version of a graduated licensing system, introduced in Austria in 1993, resulted in the incidence of crashes being reduced by more than a third (*22*). There was a probation period of two years for novice drivers and a BAC limit of 0.01 g/dl. If, during this period, there were any offences involving excess alcohol or driving that led to injury or death, a two-year extended probation was imposed, as well as obligatory attendance at a driver improvement programme.

Shaping the road network for road injury prevention

Road safety considerations are central to the planning,

design and operation of the road network. By adjusting the design of the road and road networks to accommodate human characteristics and to be more "forgiving" if an error is made, road safety engineering strategies can make a major contribution to road injury prevention and mitigation (*10*).

Safety-awareness in planning road networks

The framework for the systemic management of road safety in high-income countries is increasingly defined by the following activities (*10, 38–40*):

— classifying the road network according to their primary road functions;
— setting appropriate speed limits according to those road functions;
— improving road layout and design to encourage better use.

These approaches can, in principle, be adapted to the contexts of middle-income and low-income countries. Within these general principles, safety engineering and traffic management should aim:

— to prevent road use that does not match the functions for which the road was designed;
— to manage the traffic mix by separating different kinds of road users, so as to eliminate conflicting movements of road users, except at low speeds;
— to prevent uncertainty among road users about appropriate road use.

A large body of knowledge exists to support the use of a safety-awareness approach to road planning and is available in the form of design standards and best practice guidelines and manuals. Examples include the requirements for the development of "sustainable safety" in road networks in the Netherlands (*41*) and an earlier set of guidelines for achieving safer roads in developing countries (*10*).

Classifying roads and setting speed limits by their function

Many roads have a range of functions, and are used by different types of vehicles and by pedestrians – with large differences in speed, mass of vehicle and degree of protection. In residential areas and on urban roads this often leads to conflicts between the mobility of motor vehicle users on the one hand and the safety of pedestrians and cyclists on the other. Most pedestrian crashes occur within one mile (1.6 km) of the victim's home or place of business (*15, 42*).

Classifying roads functionally – in the form of a "road hierarchy", as it is known in highway engineering – is important for providing safer routes and safer designs. Such a classification takes account of land use, location of crash sites, vehicle and pedestrian flows, and objectives such as speed control.

The Dutch "sustainable safety" policy sets different speed limits according to the road function (see Box 4.2), together with a range of operational requirements (*41*). A study found that, by adopting these principles, a reduction of more than one third in the average number of injury crashes per million vehicle-kilometres – driven on all types of roads in the Netherlands – could be achieved (*43*).

Research is needed so that these principles can be adopted more widely, and particularly to work out how to adapt and apply them in the specific contexts of low-income countries.

Incorporating safety features into road design

A key objective of safety engineering is to make drivers naturally choose to comply with the speed limit. Through the use of self-explanatory road layouts, engineering can lead to safer road user behaviour, as well as correcting defects in road design that otherwise may lead to crashes. The following description of different types of roads illustrates the relationship between road function, road speed and road design.

Higher-speed roads

Higher-speed roads include motorways, expressways and multi-lane, divided highways with limited access. They are designed to allow for higher speeds by providing large-radius horizontal and vertical curves, "forgiving" roadsides, entry and exit "grade-separated" junctions – where there is no contact between motorized and non-motorized traffic – and median barriers to separate opposing directions of traffic. Such roads have the lowest rates of road injury in terms of distance travelled because of these design features and the fact that non-motorized users are prohibited (*39*). In low-income countries, it is also necessary to separate motorized two-wheelers from car and truck traffic travelling in the same direction.

BOX 4.2

Road types and appropriate speeds

The Dutch policy of sustainable safety divides roads into one of three types according to their function, and then sets speed limits accordingly (*41*):

- **Flow roads** (or through-roads). For such roads, through-traffic goes from the place of departure to the destination without interruption. Speeds above 100–120 km/h are not permitted, and there is a complete separation of traffic streams.
- **Distributor roads**. These roads enable users to enter or leave an area. The needs of moving traffic continue to be predominant. Local distributor roads carry traffic to and from large urban districts, villages and rural areas, and have traffic interchanges at limited sections. These roads give equal importance to motorized and non-motorized local traffic, but separate users wherever possible. Speeds on distributor roads should not exceed 50 km/h within built-up areas or 80 km/h outside such areas. There should be separate paths for pedestrians and cyclists, dual carriageways with separation of streams along the full length, speed controls at major crossings, and right of way.
- **Residential access roads**. These roads are typically used to reach a dwelling, shop or business. The needs of non-motorized users are predominant. There is a constant access and interchange of traffic and the vast majority of roads are of this type. For residential access roads in towns and villages, speeds above 30 km/h are not permitted. In rural areas, no speeds over 40 km/h are allowed at crossings and entries – otherwise 60 km/h may be acceptable.

Where a road performs a mixture of functions, the appropriate speed is normally the lowest of the speeds appropriate to the individual functions.

Single-lane carriageways

Single-lane carriageways in rural areas include many different types of road. The numbers and rates of casualties are much higher than on motorways, because of the large differences in speed between the various types of user. Crashes on local rural roads arise most commonly from vehicles leaving the road through loss of control as a result of inappropriate speed (44). Apart from speed limits, a range of engineering measures is needed to encourage appropriate speed and make hazards easily perceptible. These measures include:

— provision for slow-moving traffic and for vulnerable road users;
— lanes for overtaking, as well as lanes for vehicles waiting to turn across the path of oncoming traffic;
— median barriers to prevent overtaking and to eliminate head-on crashes;
— better highlighting of hazards through road lighting at junctions and roundabouts;
— improved vertical alignment;
— advisory speed limits at sharp bends;
— regular speed-limit signs;
— rumble strips;
— the systematic removal of roadside hazards – such as trees, utility poles and other solid objects.

Much best practice in this area has been identified in high-income countries (45).

A particular speed management problem is how to handle the transition from high-speed roads to lower-speed roads – for instance, when a vehicle leaves a motorway, or when it enters a winding stretch of narrow road after a long, straight stretch of road. The creation of transition zones on busy roads approaching towns and villages can reduce crashes and injuries for all types of road user. Design features that use a "gateway", or threshold, can influence drivers progressively to reduce their speed, and signal the beginning of the speed limit for commercial and residential areas. In approaches to slower-speed zones, rumble strips, speed humps, visual warnings in the pavement, and roundabouts have all been found useful in slowing the speed of vehicles (45). In Ghana, the introduction of rumble strips reduced crashes by some 35% and deaths by 55% in certain locations (46) (see Box 4.3).

BOX 4.3

Speed bumps in Ghana: a low-cost road safety intervention

Road safety is a serious problem in Ghana, where fatality rates are some 30 to 40 times greater than those in industrialized countries. The excessive vehicle speeds that prevail on the country's inter-urban highways and on roads in built-up areas have been shown to be a key contributory factor in serious traffic crashes (46).

In recent years, speed bumps have been installed at some crash-prone locations on the highways, so as to lower the speed of vehicles and improve the traffic environment for other road users, including pedestrians and cyclists, in built-up areas. These speed bumps produce discomfort when vehicles pass over them at higher speeds; with their vehicles lifted off the ground and with the resulting noise, drivers are forced to reduce their speed. This in turn decreases the kinetic energy of the vehicle that can cause injuries and deaths on impact, and gives drivers longer warning of possible collisions, lessening the likelihood of road crashes.

The use of speed bumps, in the form of rumble strips and speed humps, has been found to be effective on Ghanaian roads. For instance, rumble strips on the main Accra–Kumasi highway at the crash hot spot of Suhum Junction reduced the number of traffic crashes by around 35%. Fatalities fell by some 55% and serious injuries by 76%, between January 2000 and April 2001. This speed-reducing measure succeeded in reducing or even eliminating certain kinds of crashes as well as improving the safety of pedestrians (46).

Speed control bumps and humps have now become increasingly common on Ghanaian roads, particularly in built-up areas where excessive vehicle speeds threaten other road users. A wide range of materials – including vulcanized rubber, hot thermoplastic materials, bituminous mixes, concrete and bricks – have been used in the construction of the speed control areas.

Rumble strips are cheap and easy to install. They have been constructed at potentially dangerous places on the Cape Coast–Takoradi highway, the Bunso–Koforidua highway and the Tema–Akosombo highway. Speed humps, on the other hand, have been laid to slow down vehicles and improve the safety of pedestrians in the towns of Ejisu and Besease on the Accra–Kumasi highway.

Residential access roads

Residential access roads are often designed to achieve very low speeds. Speed limits, usually supported by physical self-enforcing measures to encourage compliance, are normally around 30 km/h, though lower limits are often prescribed.

Area-wide urban safety management

Engineering measures applied on an area-wide basis in towns and cities create safer conditions for pedestrians and cyclists, as well as avoiding the displacement of traffic which could lead to crashes elsewhere. Research is urgently needed in developing countries into area-wide urban safety management relating to motorized two-wheelers.

The principal road safety engineering techniques for improving the safety of pedestrians and cyclists are the provision of safer routes – through segregation and separation – and area-wide speed reduction or traffic-calming measures (22, 23). These are discussed below.

Safer routes for pedestrians and cyclists. The creation of networks of connected and convenient pedestrian and cyclist routes, together with the provision of public transport, can lead to greater safety for vulnerable road users (47). The routes will typically consist of footpaths or cycle paths separate from any carriageway, pedestrian-only areas with or without cyclists being admitted, footpaths or cycle tracks alongside carriageways, and carriageways or other surfaces shared with motor vehicles. Where pedestrian or cycle routes cross significant flows of motor vehicle traffic, the location and design of the crossing point needs special attention. Where routes are not separated from carriageways, or where space is shared with motor vehicles, the physical layout will need to manage speeds (15).

Pedestrian footpaths and pavements are used more in high-income than in low-income countries and tend to be in urban rather than rural areas. The risk of a crash on roads without pavements separating pedestrians from motorized traffic is twice that on a road with a pavement (48). Pavements in poor condition or obstructed by parked vehicles may force pedestrians to walk on the street, thus significantly increasing crash risk. This danger is particularly great for people carrying heavy loads, pushing prams, or who have difficulty in walking. Studies in low-income and middle-income countries have shown that even where pavements exist, they are often blocked – for instance, by street vendors' stalls (18, 49).

Providing pavements for pedestrians is a proven safety measure, which also helps the flow of motorized traffic. Bicycle paths have also been shown to be effective in reducing crashes, particularly at junctions (22). Danish studies have found reductions of 35% in cyclist casualties on particular routes, following the construction of cycle tracks or lanes alongside urban roads (50).

Traffic-calming measures. At speeds below 30 km/h pedestrians can coexist with motor vehicles in relative safety. Speed management and traffic-calming include techniques such as discouraging traffic from entering certain areas and installing physical speed-reducing measures, such as roundabouts, road narrowings, chicanes and road humps. These measures are often backed up by speed limits of 30 km/h, but they can be designed to achieve various levels of appropriate speed.

In Europe, there has been much experimentation with these measures and crash reductions of between 15% and 80% have been achieved (44, 51–54). In the town of Baden, Austria, about 75% of the road network is now part of a 30 km/h zone, or else a residential street with an even lower speed limit. Since integrated transport and a wide-ranging safety plan were introduced in 1988, the town has seen a 60% reduction in road casualties (55).

Most of the principles incorporated into design guidelines for traffic calming in high-income countries also apply to low-income countries, though in practice the guidelines will need to be modified because of the much higher proportion of non-motorized traffic (23). As Table 4.1, which summarizes the effects of measures undertaken in a British town, shows, area-wide speed and traffic

TABLE 4.1

Area-wide speed reduction – cost and benefits

	Town centre	Residential area
Number of road traffic injuries prevented/year	53	145
Saving-crash costs (£, 25 years, 5%[a])	33 350 000	91 260 000
Increased costs-travel time (£, 25 years, 5%[a])	21 900	53 250 000
Loss of consumers' surplus of travel[b] (£)	2 415 000	9 300 000
Total benefits (£)	9 035 000	28 710 000
Costs of implementing measures (£)	4 910 000	2 955 000
Cost–benefit	1:1.84	1:9.72

[a] 5% annual discount rate for discounting benefits to present values.
[b] Loss of benefits to consumers.

Source: reproduced from reference 56, with minor editorial amendments, with the permission of the publisher.

management can be highly effective, particularly in residential areas, where benefits have been found to exceed costs by a factor of 9.7 (56).

A systematic review of 16 controlled studies from high-income countries also showed that area-wide traffic calming in urban areas could reduce road traffic injuries. No similar studies from low-income or middle-income countries were found (57).

Safety audits

When new transport projects are proposed, area-wide safety impact assessments are needed to ensure the proposals do not have an adverse safety impact on the surrounding network. Road safety audits are then required to check that the proposed design and implementation are consistent with safety principles, and to examine whether further design changes are needed to prevent crashes (12).

The safety audit procedure is usually carried out at various stages of a new project, including:
— the feasibility study of the project;
— the draft design;
— the detailed design;
— before the project becomes operational;
— a few months after the project is operational.

An essential element of the audit process is that it should be carried out separately by both an independent design team, and a team with experience and expertise in road safety engineering and crash investigation. Guidelines for safety audits have been developed in many parts of the world, including Malaysia (58–60).

Formal safety audit procedures have been shown to be effective and cost-effective ways of improving road safety and reducing the long-term costs associated with a new road scheme (39). Mandatory safety audit procedures have existed in a number of countries including Australia, Denmark, New Zealand and the United Kingdom for several years (61). In New Zealand, it has been estimated that the procedures carry a cost–benefit ratio of 1:20 (62). A Danish study assessed the value in cost–benefit terms of 13 schemes and found first year rates of return of well over 100% (63).

Crash-protective roadsides

Collisions between vehicles leaving the road and roadside objects including trees, poles and road signs, often of very high mass, are a major road safety problem worldwide. Research that built on work by the Organisation for Economic Co-operation and Development in 1975 (64) suggests that existing strategies to tackle the problem of roadside objects would be strengthened by (65):
— designing roads without dangerous roadside objects;
— introducing a clear zone at the side of the road;
— designing roadside objects so that they are more "forgiving";
— protecting roadside objects with barriers to absorb part of the impact energy;
— protecting vehicle occupants from the consequences of collisions with roadside objects, through better vehicle design.

Collapsible lighting columns and other devices that break away on impact were first introduced in the United States in the 1970s and are now used widely throughout the world. These objects are either mounted on shear bolts, or else are constructed of a deformable, yielding material. Slip-base poles break away at the base when struck by a vehicle and include special provisions to ensure electrical safety. Early research conducted in the United States indicated that break-away columns could result in reductions in injuries of around 30% (66).

Safety barriers are frequently used to separate traffic or to prevent it from leaving the road. They are designed to deflect or contain the striking vehicle while ensuring that the forces involved do not result in serious injury to occupants of the vehicle. If properly installed and in the appropriate places, safety barriers can be effective in reducing the incidence of crashes, their severity and their consequences (67). Crash research has highlighted the need for more effective linkages between vehicle protection standards and standards for safety barriers, which take into account the range of vehicles – from small cars to heavy trucks – that are likely to make use of them.

Guard fences and rails are situated at the edge of the carriageway to deflect or contain vehicles, or in the central reserve where their aim is to reduce crashes involving vehicles crossing into approaching traffic. The fences and rails can be rigid (made of concrete), semi-rigid (made from steel beams or box beams) or flexible (made from cable or wire). Cable barriers have been used cost-effectively in Denmark, Sweden, Switzerland and the United Kingdom (65). Central cable rails are being installed to an increasing degree in Sweden to prevent dangerous overtaking on single-carriageway roads. On two-lane roads with grade-separated crossings, the use of central cable rails has produced estimated reductions of 45–50% in fatal and serious casualties (68).

Crash cushions

Crash cushions are very effective in reducing the consequences of a crash by cushioning the vehicle before it strikes rigid roadside hazards, such as bridge piers, barrier terminals, light posts and sign supports. Evaluations in the United States of crash cushion installations have found a reduc-

tion in fatal and serious injuries at crash sites of up to 75% (66). In Birmingham, England, installing crash cushions resulted in a 40% reduction in injury crashes, and a reduction (from 67% to 14%) in the number of fatal and serious crashes at the treated sites (69).

Remedial action at high-risk crash sites

The systematic implementation of low-cost road and traffic engineering measures is a highly cost-effective method of creating safer patterns of road use and correcting faults in the planning and design of the roads that have led to traffic crashes. The use of road safety audits and safety impact assessments can prevent such faults from being introduced into new or modified roads (12).

Low-cost road and traffic engineering measures consist of physical measures taken specifically to enhance the safety of the road system. Ideally, they are cheap, can be implemented quickly, and are highly cost-effective (see Table 4.2). Examples include:

— physical changes to roads to make them safer (e.g. the introduction of skid-resistant surfacing);
— the installation of central refuges and islands;
— improved lighting, signs and markings;
— changes in the operation of junctions, for example, by installing small roundabouts, changing the signal control or improving signs and markings.

Such measures can be applied at:

— high-risk sites, for instance, a particular bend or junction;
— along a section of route where the risk is greater than average, though the measures are not necessarily concentrated at specific sites;
— over a whole neighbourhood.

Experience has shown that for high benefits to be achieved relative to costs, a systematic and multidisciplinary approach to identify sites, to implement low-cost road and traffic engineering measures, and to evaluate outcomes is required, as well as an efficient organizational framework (71).

TABLE 4.2

Some examples of low-cost road safety measures in Norway			
Road safety measure	Mean cost (Norway Kroner)	Mean annual average daily traffic[a]	Cost–benefit ratio
Pedestrian bridge or underpass	5 990 000	8 765	1:2.5
Converting 3-leg junction to roundabout	5 790 000	9 094	1:1.6
Converting 4-leg junction to roundabout	4 160 000	10 432	1:2.2
Removal of roadside obstacles	310 000	20 133	1:19.3
Minor improvements (miscellaneous)	5 640 000	3 269	1:1.5
Guard rail along roadside	860 000	10 947	1:10.4
Median guard rail	1 880 000	42 753	1:10.3
Signing of hazardous curves	60 000	1 169	1:3.5
Road lighting	650 000	8 179	1:10.7
Upgrading marked pedestrian crossings	390 000	10 484	1:14.0

[a] The sum of all motor vehicles passing a point on the road in a single year, divided by 365; this value excludes pedestrians and cyclists.

Source: reproduced from reference *70*, with minor editorial amendments, with the permission of the author.

Providing visible, crash-protective, "smart" vehicles

Improving the visibility of vehicles

Daytime running lights for cars

The term, "daytime running lights" refers to the use of lights (whether multipurpose or specially designed) on the front of a vehicle while it is running during daylight hours, so as to increase its visibility. Some countries – including Austria, Canada, Hungary, the Nordic countries and some states in the United States – now require by law varying levels of use of daytime running lights (*16*). This may involve either drivers switching on their headlamps or the fitting of switches or special lamps on vehicles.

Two meta-analyses of the effects of daytime running lights on cars show that the measure contributes substantially to reducing road crashes. The first study, which examined daytime crashes involving more than one party, found a reduction in the number of crashes of around 13% with the use of daytime lights, and reduction of between 8% and 15% as a result of introducing mandatory laws on daytime use (*16*). The number of pedestrians and cyclists hit by cars was reduced by 15% and 10%, respectively. The second study found a reduction of slightly over 12% in daytime crashes involving more than one party, a 20% decrease in injured victims and a 25% reduction in deaths in such crashes (*72*). A study of data over four years from nine American

states concluded that, on average, cars fitted with automatic daytime running lights were involved in 3.2% fewer multiple crashes than vehicles without (*73*). Following the introduction of daytime running lights and the enforcement of their use in Hungary, there has been a 13% reduction in the number of frontal crashes in daylight (*74*).

A cost–benefit analysis of providing automatic light switches on cars for daytime running lamps using standard low-beam headlights found that the benefits outweighed the costs by a factor of 4.4. The fitting of daytime running lights with special lamps with economical bulbs increased the cost–benefit to a factor of 6.4 (*75*). Motorized two-wheeler users have expressed concerns that daytime running lights on cars could reduce the visibility of motorcyclists. While there is no empirical evidence to indicate this is the case, researchers have suggested that if such an effect did exist, it would be offset by the benefit to motorcyclists of increased car visibility (*22, 72*). In the two meta-analyses cited above, use of car daytime running lamps led to a reduction in pedestrian and cyclist crashes (*16, 72*).

High-mounted stop lamps in cars

High-mounted stop lamps on cars have also been adopted as standard equipment in many countries. They have led to a reduction of between 15% and 50% in rear crashes and cost–benefit ratios of 1:4.1 in Norway and 1:8.9 in the United States (*16*).

Daytime running lights for motorized two-wheelers

The use of daytime running lights by motorized two-wheelers has been shown to reduce visibility-related crashes in several countries by between 10% and 15%. In a study of 14 states in the United States with motorcycle headlight-use laws, a 13% reduction in fatal daytime crashes was observed (76). In Singapore, a study conducted 14 months after the introduction of legislation requiring motorcyclists to switch on their headlamps found that fatal daytime crashes had reduced by 15% (77). In Malaysia, where legislation requiring daytime use was preceded by a two-month information campaign, the number of visibility-related crashes fell by 29% (78). In Europe, motorcyclists who use daytime running lights have a crash rate that is about 10% lower than that of motorcyclists who do not (22).

One estimate of the cost–benefit ratio of using running lights in daytime is put at around 1:5.4 for mopeds and 1:7.2 for motorcycles (16).

Improving the visibility of non-motorized vehicles

The main intervention for pedestrians to protect themselves is to wear clothing that increases their visibility, especially in poor daylight and in darkness. For cyclists, front, rear and wheel reflectors, and bicycle lamps that are visible at specified distances, are often required in high-income countries. The quality and use of lights can be improved by enabling the storage of separate light systems or by designing the lighting into the cycle frame (15).

Safety researchers in low-income countries have suggested various means for improving the visibility of vulnerable road users. The use of retro-reflective vests, common in high-income countries, may be problematic owing to their cost and the discomfort in wearing them in hot climates. A design for a brightly-coloured orange or yellow shopping bag that can quickly be transformed into a conspicuous vest has been proposed for two-wheeler users in low-income countries (79). Encouraging the use of colours such as orange and yellow for bicycles, for wheels, and for the rear ends of rickshaws and other non-motorized vehicles, has also been suggested (23).

Many countries require the fitting of reflectors on the front and rear of non-motorized vehicles. In low-income countries, though, rules could be extended to cover all animal carts, cycle trishaws and other forms of local transport that currently create road safety risks because of their poor visibility at night. The use of reflectors on the sides of vehicles may be helpful at junctions (23). However, while all these aids to visibility would appear to have great potential, their actual effectiveness in increasing the safety of pedestrians and cyclists remains largely unknown and requires additional study (80).

Crash-protective vehicle design

While market forces can help advance in-car safety in individual car models, the aim of harmonizing legislative standards of vehicle design is to ensure a uniform and acceptable level of safety across a whole product line.

Legislative standards are produced by different authorities, from the national to international level. On a global scale, these include the United Nations Economic Commission for Europe, and on a regional level, groupings such as the European Union. Standardization at the regional and national levels, taking into account as it does local conditions, can often produce faster action than a similar process at the international level. High-income countries routinely set out their national priorities in reports to the International Technical Conferences on the Enhanced Safety of Vehicles. Priorities in some low-income and middle-income countries have also been identified (23, 81–83).

A study in the United Kingdom concluded that improved vehicle crash protection (also known as "secondary safety" or "passive safety") for car occupants and pedestrians would have the greatest effect, out of all new policies under consideration, in reducing road casualties in Great Britain (see Table 4.3) (84). Comparable analyses in New Zealand estimated that improvements being made in the safety of the vehicle fleet would reduce projected social costs in 2010 by just under 16% (85).

TABLE 4.3

Estimated serious and fatal road casualty reduction effects of new policies, averaged over all types of roads, for different road users, United Kingdom (expressed a percentage reduction in the number of road casualties)

Policy	Car occupants	Pedestrians	Cyclists	Motorcyclists	Others	All users
New road safety engineering programme	6.0	13.7	4.3	6.0	6.0	7.7
Improved vehicle crash protection (passive safety)	10.0	15.0	—	—	—	8.6
Other vehicle safety improvements	5.4	2.0	3.2	8.0	3.0	4.6
Motorcycle and bicycle helmets	—	—	6.0	7.0	—	1.4
Improving safety of rural single carriageways	4.1	—	—	4.2	4.1	3.4
Reducing crash involvement of novice drivers	2.8	1.3	1.0	0.8	0.4	1.9
Additional measures for pedestrians and cyclist protection	—	6.0	4.0	—	—	1.2
Additional measures for speed reduction	5.0	5.0	5.0	5.0	5.0	5.0
Additional measures for child protection	—	6.9	0.6	—	—	1.7
Reducing casualties in drink-drive accidents	1.9	0.4	0.2	0.8	0.5	1.2
Reducing crashes during high-mileage work driving	2.1	0.9	1.2	1.9	1.9	1.9
Additional measures for improved driver behaviour	1.0	1.0	1.0	1.0	1.0	1.0
Combined effect of all measures	33	42	24	30	19	35

Source: reproduced from reference *84*, with minor editorial amendments, with the permission of the publisher.

The concept of "crashworthiness" in vehicle design is now well understood and is incorporated into current car design in highly-motorized countries. If it were adopted globally, it would contribute substantially to increased road safety (*82*) (see Box 4.4).

Safer car fronts to protect pedestrians and cyclists

The majority of fatally-injured pedestrians are hit by the fronts of cars. Creating safer car fronts is thus a key means of improving pedestrian safety (*26, 88, 89*).

Crash engineers have known for some time how crash-protection techniques can be used to reduce deaths and serious injuries to pedestrians struck by the fronts of cars (*90–93*). Since the late 1970s, studies have been conducted on how the shape, stiffness and speed of passenger cars influence the

---

BOX 4.4

Vehicle safety standards

Vehicle engineering for improved safety can be achieved by modifying a vehicle to help the driver avoid a crash, or in the event of a crash, protect both those inside and outside the car against injury.

Research indicates that vehicle crash protection is a most effective strategy for reducing death and serious injury in road crashes. A review of the effectiveness of casualty reduction measures in the United Kingdom between 1980 and 1996 found that the greatest contribution to reducing casualties was secondary safety or crash protection improvements to vehicles. These accounted for around 15% of the reduction, compared with 11% for drink-drive measures and 6.5% for road safety engineering measures (*84*).

Another review, by the European Transport Safety Council, estimated that improved standards for crash protection could reduce deaths and serious injuries on European roads by as much as 20% (*86*). Analysis has shown that if all cars were designed to provide impact protection equivalent to that of the best cars in the same class, half of all fatal and disabling injuries could be avoided (*87*).

During the 1990s, significant steps towards improved protection of occupants of cars were made in the highly-motorized countries. In the European Union, there were several directives on frontal and side impact protection, and information on crash tests from the European New Car Assessment Programme (EuroNCAP) was widely disseminated. Much of the research and development necessary for improvements in other safety areas for car occupants – such as smart seat-belt reminders – has been completed and now requires legislation to bring it into force.

Globally, the predominant category of road casualties up to 2020 will continue to be vulnerable road users. Protection for those outside the vehicle against impact is thus a priority in the field of vehicle design.

resulting injuries of pedestrians and pedal cyclists. While the fitting of rigid, "aggressive" bull-bars has been much publicized as a cause for concern, research shows that it is, in fact, the ordinary car front that presents by far the greatest risk to pedestrians and cyclists in a frontal impact (*93–95*).

Performance requirements and test procedures have been devised by a consortium established by European governments – the European Enhanced Vehicle-safety Committee (EEVC). Between 1988 and 1994, an EEVC working group on pedestrian protection developed a complete series of test methods to evaluate the front of passenger cars with respect to pedestrian safety (*92*), and these test methods were further improved in 1998 (*95*). The tests assume an impact speed of 40 km/h and consist of the following:

— a bumper test to prevent serious knee-joint injuries and leg fractures;
— a bonnet leading-edge test to prevent femur and hip fractures in adults and head injuries in children;
— two tests involving the bonnet top to prevent life-threatening head injuries.

It has been estimated that take up of these tests could avoid 20% of deaths and serious injuries to pedestrians and cyclists in European Union countries annually (*87, 94, 96*).

These tests, with minor amendments have been used by the European New Car Assessment Programme since 1997, and more recently by the Australian New Car Assessment Programme. Of the many new cars tested to date, only one type of car has shown evidence of having reasonable protection – about 80% of the protection demanded by the tests at an estimated additional manufacturing cost for new designs of €10 per car (*97*). Studies carried out by national road safety research organizations in Europe have shown that the benefits of adopting the four EEVC tests would outweigh the costs (*98*).

Legislation in this area is expected shortly in several countries, but the contents of the legislation are the subject of continuing international discussions (*87, 99*). Experts believe that the adoption of the well-researched EEVC tests would save many

lives (*82, 93, 100*) – perhaps as many as 2000 lives annually in the European Union alone (*87*).

Safer bus and truck fronts

Extending the crash-protective vehicle exterior concept to vans, pick-up trucks and other trucks, and buses is an urgent requirement for protecting vulnerable road users in low-income countries (*82, 88, 101*). Buses and trucks are involved in a greater proportion of crashes in low-income countries than they are in high-income countries (*102*). Preliminary investigations have suggested that significant reductions in injuries could be achieved if the geometry and design of truck fronts were changed (*102*). The critical geometric features that influence injury and that continue to require attention by truck designers have been set out (*101*). Given the growth of megacities such as Bangkok, Beijing, Mexico City, São Paulo, Shanghai and others, the protection of vulnerable road users from bus and truck fronts take on particular importance. Many such cities have unique vehicles, such as the *tuk-tuk* of Bangkok, the *becak* of Jakarta and the three-wheeled taxis of India. Such vehicles incorporate almost no concept of crash protection, for either pedestrians or occupants. They present a good opportunity, therefore, for technical knowledge to improve their safety to be transferred from western car designers (*23*).

Car occupant protection

The essential aims in crash protection are:

— to maintain, through appropriate design, the integrity of the car's passenger compartment;
— to provide protection against elements that could cause injury in the car's interior;
— to ensure that vehicle occupants are appropriately restrained;
— to reduce the probability of an occupant being ejected;
— to prevent injury to other occupants (in a frontal crash, unbelted rear-seat occupants can cause injury to belted occupants seated in front of them);
— to improve the compatibility between vehicles of different mass (e.g. between car and

sports utility vehicle, car and car, car and bus or truck, car and motorized two-wheeler or bicycle).

Car crash protection standards currently address areas such as structural design, and the design and fitting of seat-belts, child restraints, air bags, anti-burst door latches, laminated glass windscreens, seats, and head restraints. Such standards offering a minimum, but high level of protection need to be adopted in all countries.

Frontal and side impact protection. The vast majority of car crashes in high-income countries are offset frontal crashes (where only one side of a vehicle's front end hits the other vehicle or object). In the United States, for example, 79% of injuries from frontal crashes occur as a result of offset frontal crashes (*81*). A recent priority for safety engineers working on frontal impact protection has been to improve the car structure so it can endure severe offset impacts with little or no intrusion of external objects. This allows space, in the event of a crash, for the seat-belts and air bags to slow down the occupants with the minimum risk of injury.

In most high-income countries, there are legislative performance requirements for cars to undergo a full-width frontal barrier test or an off-set deformable barrier test. The former is acknowl-edged as an appropriate method for testing occu-pant restraint systems in frontal crashes. The latter, the offset deformable barrier test, is a more realistic simulation of what happens to a car's structure in a typical injury-producing frontal crash. The use of both tests is therefore important to ensure crash protection for car occupants (*83, 103*). Both tests are appropriate for more types of vehicle than they are currently used for.

Side impacts, while less frequent than frontal crashes, typically cause more severe injuries. In side impacts, it is difficult to prevent occupants on the side that is struck from coming into contact with the car's interior. Attempts at greater protection thus rely on managing the problem of intrusion, and providing padding and side air bags. During the 1990s, legislative standards were introduced in most high-income countries to offer better protec-tion in side impacts. Following the experiences and evaluation of these requirements for frontal and side impact protection in Europe, various improve-ments have since been identified (*83, 104*).

As mentioned earlier, advanced crash tests, car-ried out for the benefit of consumer information by various New Car Assessment Programmes and by organizations such as the Insurance Institute for Highway Safety in the United States, play a vital role in promoting car design that provides good frontal and side impact protection.

Occupant restraints. The use of seat-belts con-tinues to be the most important form of occupant restraint. Measures to increase their use – by means of legislation, information, enforcement and smart audible seat-belt reminders – are central to improving the safety of car occupants. When used, seat-belts have been found to reduce the risk of serious and fatal injury by between 40% and 65%. The fitting of anchorages and seat-belts are covered by various technical standards worldwide and in most countries these standards are mandatory for cars. However, there is anec-dotal evidence that a half or more of all vehicles in low-income countries may lack functioning seat-belts (*17*).

Air bags are being increasingly provided in cars as an extra means of restraint, in addition to three-point seat-belts. They should be fitted universally to increase the protection of occupants involved in crashes. While driver and front-seat passenger air bags do not offer protection in all types of impact and do not diminish the risk of ejection (*105*), when combined with seat-belt use, they have been found to reduce the risk of death in frontal crashes by 68% (*106*). Estimates of the general effectiveness of air bags in reducing deaths in all types of crashes range from 8% to 14% (*106–108*). Where passenger air bags are fitted, however, clear instructions are needed to avoid fitting rear-facing child restraints on the same seat. Also required are devices to auto-matically detect child restraints and out-of-posi-tion occupants, and in such cases to switch off the passenger air bag.

Protection against roadside objects. Collisions between cars and trees or poles are characterized by the severity of the injuries produced. Current legislation only requires the use of crash tests with barriers representing car-to-car impacts. It may now be time to supplement these tests with front and side car-to-pole tests, as practised in some consumer testing programmes. Better coordination is required between the design of cars and that of safety barriers (*65, 109*).

Vehicle-to-vehicle compatibility

Achieving vehicle-to-vehicle compatibility in crashes depends upon the particular mix of motor vehicle. In the United States, for example, there is a greater need to reconcile sports utility vehicles and other light truck vehicles with passenger cars. The United States National Highway Traffic Safety Administration has made vehicle compatibility one of its leading priorities and has published its proposed initiatives in a recent report (*110*). In Europe, work focuses on trying to improve car-to-car compatibility for both front-to-front and front-to-side crashes and recommendations on this have been put forward (*83*). In low-income and middle-income countries, issues of vehicle-to-vehicle compatibility are related more to collisions between cars and trucks − both front-to-front impacts, as well as between the front of the car and the rear of the truck. The first priority for these countries must be to improve the geometry and structure of trucks so as to better accommodate impacts from smaller vehicles − not only cars, but motorcycles and bicycles as well (*82*).

The frontal structures of many new cars are capable of absorbing their own kinetic energy in crashes, so avoiding any significant intrusion of the passenger compartment. However, there is currently no legal control, by means of performance requirements, of the relative degrees of stiffness of the fronts of different models of car. Consequently, when cars of differing stiffness collide, the stiffer car crushes the weaker car (*83*).

Front, rear and side under-run guards on trucks

The provision of front and rear under-run protection on trucks is a well-established means of pre-venting "under-running" by cars (whereby cars go underneath trucks, because of a mismatch between the heights of car fronts and truck sides and fronts). Similarly, side protection prevents cyclists from being run over. It has been estimated that the provision of energy-absorbing front, rear and side under-run protection could reduce deaths by about 12% (*111*). It has also been suggested that the benefits would exceed the costs, even if the safety effect of these measures was as low as 5% (*56*).

Design of non-motorized vehicles

Research has shown that ergonomic changes in the design of bicycles could lead to an improvement in bicycle safety (*23, 112*). Bicycles display large differences in component strength and the reliability of their brakes and lighting. About three quarters of crashes involving passengers carried on bicycles in the Netherlands are associated with feet being trapped in the wheel spokes, and 60% of bicycles have no protective system to prevent this (*112*).

"Intelligent" vehicles

New technologies are creating new opportunities for road safety as more intelligent systems are being developed for road vehicles. Vehicles are now starting to be equipped with technology that could improve road safety in terms of exposure, crash avoidance, injury reduction and automatic post-crash notification of collision (*113*).

The development of intelligent systems is principally technology-driven. This means that − in the case of many of the features being promoted − the implications for road safety, as well as for the behavioural response of users and for public acceptance, have to be examined. It is generally acknowledged that some devices may distract drivers or affect their behaviour, often in a manner not anticipated by the designers of the system (*113, 114*). For these and other reasons, it has been strongly suggested that the development and application of intelligent transport systems should not be left entirely to market forces (*87, 113*).

Examples are presented below of some of the most promising "intelligent" vehicle safety applications that are already "on the road" in some form.

"Smart", audible seat-belt reminders

As discussed earlier, the fitting and use of seat-belts constitute the most important form of occupant restraint. Measures to increase seat-belt use, through legislation, information and enforcement and smart audible seat-belt reminders are central to improving in-car safety.

Seat-belt reminders are intelligent visual and audible devices that detect whether seat-belts are in use in various seating positions and give out increasingly urgent warning signals until the belts are used (*83*). They do not lock the ignition function. Modern types of seat-belt reminders are different from the older versions that produced a chiming sound and a light for four to eight seconds, which proved ineffective in increasing seat-belt use (*115*).

In Sweden, 35% of all new cars sold currently have seat-belt reminders (*116*). It is estimated in that country that reminders in all cars could lead to national levels of seat-belt use of around 97%, contributing to a reduction of some 20% in car occupant deaths (*117*).

User trials and research in Sweden and the United States have shown that seat-belt reminders with audible warnings are an effective means of increasing seat-belt use. Preliminary research on the only system currently available in the United States found a 7% increase in seat-belt use among drivers of cars with seat-belt reminders, compared with drivers of unequipped vehicles (*118*). Furthermore, a driver survey found that of the two thirds who activated the system, three quarters reported using their seat-belt, and nearly half of all respondents said their belt use had increased (*119*).

A recent United States National Academy of Science report urged the car industry to ensure that every new light-duty vehicle should have, as standard equipment, an enhanced seat-belt reminder system for front-seat occupants, with an audible warning and visual indicator that could not be easily disconnected (*120*).

An Australian analysis has estimated a cost–benefit ratio of 1:5, for a simple device for drivers only (*121*). A cost–benefit ratio of 1:6 was found when seat-belt reminders were introduced in new vehicles in European Union countries (*75*). Seat-belt reminders provide a cheap and efficient option for helping to enforce seat-belt use.

Speed adaptation

As stated elsewhere in this report, a variety of effective means exist to reduce vehicle speeds – including the setting of speed limits according to road function, better road design, and the enforcement of limits by the police, radar and speed cameras. Speed limitation devices in vehicles can assist this process, by controlling the maximum speed a vehicle can travel at; some devices are able to set variable limits (see below).

Insurance statistics show that high-speed cars – those with powerful engines, high acceleration and high top speeds – are more frequently involved in crashes than cars with lower speed capacities (*16*). The increase in maximum speeds in the past 30 to 40 years has made it increasingly easy to drive at inappropriately fast speeds, thus countering the effects of measures aimed at improving the safety of cars. In 1993, the ten best-selling models of cars had top speeds that were double the highest national posted speed limits in Norway (*16*).

Intelligent Speed Adaptation (ISA) is a system being developed that shows great promise in terms of its potential impact on the incidence of road casualties. With this system, the vehicle "knows" the permitted or recommended maximum speed for the road along which it is travelling.

The standard system uses an in-vehicle digital road map onto which speed limits have been coded, combined with a satellite positioning system. The level at which the system intervenes to control the speed of the vehicle can be one of the following:

— advisory – the driver is informed of the speed limit and when it is being exceeded;
— voluntary – the system is linked to the vehicle controls but the driver can choose whether and when to override it;
— mandatory – no override of the system is possible.

The potential reduction in the number of fatal crashes for these different types of systems has been estimated to be in the range 18–25% for advisory systems, 19–32% for voluntary systems, and 37–59% for mandatory systems (*122*). Speed limit information can in theory be extended to incorporate lower speeds at certain locations in the network and – in the future – can vary according to current network conditions, such as weather conditions, traffic density and the presence of traffic incidents on the road.

Experimental trials have been carried out or are under way in Australia, Denmark, the Netherlands, Sweden and the United Kingdom (*113*). By far the largest trial of a speed adaptation system – the three-year Intelligent Speed Adaptation project – was carried out in four municipalities in Sweden. Various types of ISA system were installed in around 5000 cars, buses and trucks. If the driver exceeded the speed limit, light and sound signals were activated. The trial was conducted primarily in built-up areas with speed limits of 50 km/h or 30 km/h, and the test drivers were both private car and commercial drivers. The Swedish National Road Administration reported a high level of driver acceptance in urban areas of the devices and suggested that they could reduce crash injuries by 20–30% in urban areas (*109, 116*).

Alcohol interlocks

Alcohol ignition interlocks are automatic control systems that are designed to prevent drivers who are persistently over the legal alcohol limit from starting their cars if their BAC levels are over the legal driving limit. In principle, these devices can be fitted in any car. As a deterrent, though, they can be fitted in the cars of repeat drink-driving offenders, who have to blow into the device before the car will start. If the driver's BAC is above a certain level, the car will not start. Such devices, when introduced in vehicles as part of a comprehensive monitoring programme, led to reductions of between 40% and 95% in the rate of repeated offending (*123*).

Around half of Canada's provinces and territories have embarked on alcohol interlock programmes and in the United States, most states have passed enabling legislation for such devices. Some states in Australia have small experimental programmes

in progress, involving public transport and commercial road transport, and the European Union is conducting a feasibility study (*124*). In Sweden, alcohol interlocks are now installed in over 1500 vehicles and, since 2002, two major truck suppliers have been offering interlocks as standard equipment on the Swedish market (*116*).

If limited to use in dealing with drivers who are persistently over the legal alcohol limit, alcohol interlock devices might have only a numerically small impact. However, their wider use in public and commercial transport in the future could extend the potential impact of this tool in dealing with the problem of drink-driving.

On-board electronic stability programmes

Weather conditions can affect the control of vehicles and increase the risk of skidding and crashes due to loss of control on wet or icy roads. In such conditions an electronic stability programme – an on-board car safety system – can help the car to remain stable during critical manoeuvring. Such devices are now being introduced onto the market, but they are very expensive. A recent Swedish evaluation of the effects of this new technology – the first of its kind – produced promising results, especially for bad weather conditions, with reductions in injury crashes of 32% and 38% on ice and snow, respectively (*125*).

Setting and securing compliance with key road safety rules

Good enforcement is an integral part of road safety. Self-enforcing road safety engineering measures, as well as new and existing vehicle technologies that influence the behaviour of road users have already been discussed. This section examines the role of traffic law enforcement by the police and the use of camera technology.

A major review on traffic law enforcement identified several important findings (*126*):

- It is critical that the deterrent be meaningful for the traffic law enforcement to be successful.
- Enforcement levels need to be high and maintained over a period of time, so as to ensure that the perceived risk of being caught remains high.

- Once offenders are caught, their penalties should be dealt with swiftly and efficiently.
- Using selective enforcement strategies to target particular risk behaviours and choosing specific locations both improve the effectiveness of enforcement.
- Of all the methods of enforcement, automated means – such as cameras – are the most cost-effective.
- Publicity supporting enforcement measures increases their effectiveness; used on its own, publicity has a negligible effect on road user behaviour.

A study in Canada found that the enforcement of traffic rules reduced the frequency of fatal motor vehicle crashes in highly-motorized countries. At the same time, inadequate or inconsistent enforcement could contribute to thousands of deaths worldwide every year (*127*). It has been estimated that if all current cost-effective traffic law enforcement strategies were rigorously applied by European Union countries, then as many as 50% of deaths and serious injuries in these countries might be prevented (*128*).

Setting and enforcing speed limits

Setting road speed limits is closely associated with road function and road design, as already mentioned. Physical measures related to the road and the vehicle, as well as law enforcement by the police, all contribute to ensuring compliance with maximum posted speed limits and to the choice of an appropriate speed for the existing conditions.

Much research and international experience point to the effectiveness of setting and enforcing speed limits in reducing the frequency and severity of road crashes (*16, 129*). Some examples of the impacts of changes in speed limits are given in Table 4.4. In addition, the use of variable speed limits – where different speed limits are imposed at different times on the same stretch of road – can be effective in managing speed (*128, 130*).

Speed enforcement on rural roads

A meta-analysis of speed enforcement on rural roads, either by means of radar or instruments which measure mean vehicle speed between two fixed points, or by stationary speed enforcement – where uniformed police officers and police cars attend vehicle stopping points – found that the two strategies combined reduced fatal crashes by 14% and injury crashes by 6%. Stationary speed enforcement alone reduced fatal and injury crashes by 6% (*16*).

Leggett described a long-term, low-intensity speed enforcement strategy in Tasmania, Australia, that involved the visible use of single, stationary police vehicles on three high-risk stretches of rural road (*131*). This enforcement strategy resulted in an observed reduction in speeding behaviour and a significant decrease in the overall average speed of 3.6 km/h. A fall of 58% in serious casualty crashes – fatal crashes and those involving hospital admission – was also reported. The two-year enforcement programme produced an estimated cost–benefit ratio of 1:4 (*131*).

TABLE 4.4

Examples of effects of speed limit changes					
Date	Country	Type of road	Speed limit change	Effect of change on speed	Effect of change on number of fatalities
1985	Switzerland	Motorways	130 km/h to 120 km/h	5 km/h decrease in mean speeds	12% reduction
1985	Switzerland	Rural roads	100 km/h to 80 km/h	10 km/h decrease in mean speeds	6% reduction
1985	Denmark	Roads in built-up areas	60 km/h to 50 km/h	3–4 km/h decrease in mean speeds	24% reduction
1987	USA	Interstate highways	55 miles/h (88.5 km/h) to 65 miles/h (104.6 km/h)	2–4 miles/h (3.2–6.4 km/h) increase in mean speeds	19–34% increase
1989	Sweden	Motorways	110 km/h to 90 km/h	14.4 km/h decrease in median speeds	21% reduction

Source: reproduced from reference *130,* with the permission of the publisher.

Speed cameras

Automatic speed enforcement, such as by means of speed cameras, is now employed in many countries. Experience from a range of high-income countries indicates that speed cameras that record photographic evidence of a speeding offence, that is admissible in a law court, are a highly effective means of speed enforcement (see Table 4.5). The well-publicized use of such equipment in places where speed limits are not generally obeyed and where the consequent risk of a crash is high has led to substantial reductions in crashes (113, 132, 134). The cost–benefit ratios of speed cameras have been reported to range between 1:3 and 1:27 (135, 136). In several countries, including Finland, Norway and the United Kingdom, there has been a high social acceptance of speed cameras (113).

Speed limiters in heavy goods and public transport vehicles

Speed can also be controlled by "vehicle speed limiters" or "speed governors", which are devices that can be added to vehicles to limit the maximum speed of the vehicle. This device is already being used in many countries in heavy goods vehicles and coaches. It has been estimated that speed governors on heavy goods vehicles could contribute to a reduction of 2% in the total number of injury crashes (137).

In rural areas, speed limitation for buses, minibuses and trucks could be valuable (46). Given the high representation of such vehicles in injury crashes in low-income countries, universal availability of speed limitation on trucks and buses would be an important means of improving road safety.

Setting and enforcing alcohol impairment laws

Despite the progress made in many countries in curbing drink-driving, alcohol is still a significant and widespread factor in road crashes. The scientific literature and national road safety programmes agree that a package of effective measures is necessary to reduce alcohol-related crashes and injuries.

Blood alcohol concentration limits

The basic element of any package to reduce alcohol impairment among road users is establishing a legal BAC limit. In many countries, a breath alcohol limit is used, for purposes of legal prosecution. Mandatory BAC limits provide an objective and simple means by which alcohol impairment can be detected (138). In addition, the BAC level gives clear guidance to drivers about safe driving practice. Upper limits of 0.05 g/dl for the general driving population and 0.02 g/dl for young drivers and motorcycle riders are generally considered to be the best practice at this time.

TABLE 4.5

Estimated safety benefits of speed cameras

Country or area	Benefits of crash reduction at a system level	Benefits of crash reduction at individual crash sites
Australia	22% reduction in all crashes in New South Wales 30% reduction in all crashes on urban arterial roads in Victoria 34% reduction in fatal crashes in Queensland	
New Zealand		11% reduction in crashes and 20% reduction in casualties during trials of hidden speed cameras
Republic of Korea		28% reduction in crashes and 60% reduction in deaths at high-risk sites
United Kingdom		35% reduction in road traffic deaths and serious injuries and 56% reduction in pedestrians killed or seriously injured at camera site
Europe (various)	50% reduction in all crashes	
Various countries (meta-analysis)	17% reduction in crashes resulting in injuries 28% reduction in all crashes in urban areas 4% reduction in all crashes in rural areas	

Sources: references 16, 113, 132, 133.

Blood alcohol concentration limits for the general driving population

The risk of crash involvement starts to increase significantly at BAC levels of 0.04 g/dl (*139*). A variety of BAC limits are in place across the world – ranging from 0.02 g/dl to 0.10 g/dl (see Table 4.6). The most common limit in high-income countries is 0.05 g/dl; a legal limit of 0.10 g/dl corresponds to a three-fold increase, and a limit of 0.08 g/dl a two-fold increase, in the risk of crash involvement over that allowed by a 0.05 g/dl limit.

Reviews of the effectiveness of introducing BAC limits for the first time have found that they lead to reductions in alcohol-related crashes, though the magnitude of these effects varies considerably. When limits are subsequently decreased, research shows that this is generally accompanied by further reductions in alcohol-related crashes, injuries and deaths (*138*). Reducing BAC limits from 0.10 g/dl to 0.08 g/dl (as was done in some states in the United States) or from 0.08 g/dl to 0.05 g/dl (in Australia) or from 0.05 g/dl to 0.02 g/dl (in Sweden) resulted in a fall in the number of deaths and serious injuries (*143–145*). In the United States, a systematic review of BAC laws in 16 states found that the reduction from 0.10 g/dl to 0.08 g/dl resulted in a median decrease of 7% in fatal alcohol-related motor vehicle crashes (*145*).

Lower blood alcohol concentration limits for young or inexperienced drivers

As already discussed in the previous chapter, the crash risk for inexperienced young adults starts to increase substantially at lower BAC levels than older, more experienced drivers.

A review of published studies found that laws establishing a lower BAC limit – of between zero and 0.02 g/dl – for young or inexperienced drivers

TABLE 4.6

Blood alcohol concentration (BAC) limits for drivers by country or area

Country or area	BAC (g/dl)	Country or area	BAC (g/dl)
Australia	0.05	Lesotho	0.08
Austria	0.05	Luxembourg	0.05
Belgium	0.05	Netherlands	0.05
Benin	0.08	New Zealand	0.08
Botswana	0.08	Norway	0.05
Brazil	0.08	Portugal	0.05
Canada	0.08	Russian Federation	0.02
Côte d'Ivoire	0.08	South Africa	0.05
Czech Republic	0.05	Spain	0.05
Denmark	0.05	Swaziland	0.08
Estonia	0.02	Sweden	0.02
Finland	0.05	Switzerland	0.08
France	0.05	Uganda	0.15
Germany	0.05	United Kingdom	0.08
Greece	0.05	United Republic of Tanzania	0.08
Hungary	0.05	United States of America[a]	0.10 or 0.08
Ireland	0.08	Zambia	0.08
Italy	0.05	Zimbabwe	0.08
Japan	0.00		

[a] Depends on state legislation.
Sources: references *140–142*.

can lead to reductions in crashes of between 4% and 24% (*145*). In the United States, where a lower BAC limit applies to all drivers under the age of 21 years, it has been estimated that the cost–benefit ratio of the measure is 1:11 (*146*). In other countries, there are lower legal BAC limits for newly-licensed drivers, or for newly-licensed drivers under a certain age, which form part of a graduated driver licensing scheme.

Minimum drinking-age laws

Minimum drinking-age laws specify an age below which the purchase or public consumption of alcoholic beverages is illegal. In the United States, the minimum drinking age in all 50 states is currently 21 years. A systematic review of 14 studies from various countries looking at the effects of raising minimum drinking ages found that crash-related outcomes decreased on average by 16% for the targeted age groups. In nine studies that examined the effects of lowering the drinking-age, crash-related outcomes increased by an average of 10% within the age groups concerned (*145*).

Deterring excess alcohol offenders

For most countries, the level of enforcement of drink-driving laws has a direct effect on the incidence of drinking and driving (*147*). Increasing drivers' perception of the risk of being detected is the most effective means of deterring drinking and driving (*148*). "Evidential" breath-testing devices (devices that are considered accurate enough for the results to be used as evidence in law courts) are a means of substantially increasing breath-testing activity. Though used in most high-income countries, they are not currently widespread elsewhere. This greatly limits the ability of many countries to respond effectively to the problem of drink-driving.

The deterrent effect of breath-testing devices is to a large extent dependent on the legislation governing their use (*126*). Police powers vary between countries, and include the following:

— stopping obviously impaired drivers;
— stopping drivers at roadblocks or sobriety checkpoints and testing only those suspected of alcohol impairment;
— stopping drivers at random and testing all who are stopped.

The following components have been identified as being central to successful police enforcement operations to deter drinking drivers (*128*):

• A high proportion of people tested (at least one in ten drivers every year but, if possible, one in three drivers, as is the case in Finland). This can only be achieved through wide-scale application of random breath testing and evidential breath testing.
• Enforcement that is unpredictable in terms of time and place, deployed in such a manner so as to ensure wide coverage of the whole road network and to make it difficult for drivers to avoid the checkpoints.
• Highly visible police operations. For drinking drivers who are caught, remedial treatment can be offered as an alternative to traditional penalties, to reduce the likelihood of repeated offending.

Random breath testing and sobriety checkpoints

Random breath testing is carried out in several countries, including Australia, Colombia, France, the Nordic countries, the Netherlands, New Zealand and South Africa. The use of sustained and intensive random breath testing is a highly effective means of reducing injuries resulting from alcohol impairment. In Australia, for instance, since 1993 it has led to estimated reductions in alcohol-related deaths in New South Wales of 36% (with one in three drivers tested), in Tasmania of 42% (three in four tested) and in Victoria of 40% (one in two tested) (*126*).

An international review of the effectiveness of random breath testing and sobriety checkpoints found that both reduced alcohol-related crashes by about 20% (*149*). The reductions appeared to be similar, irrespective of whether the checkpoints were used for short-term intensive campaigns or continuously over a period of several years.

A Swiss study has shown that random breath testing is one of the most cost-effective safety measures that can be employed, with a cost–benefit ratio estimated at 1:19 (*150*). In New South Wales, Australia, the estimated cost–benefit ratio of random breath testing ranged from 1:1 to 1:56 (*126, 151, 152*). Similarly, economic analyses on the sobriety checkpoint programmes in the United States estimated benefits totalling between 6 and 23 times their original cost (*153, 154*).

Mass media campaigns

It is generally accepted that enforcement of alcohol impairment laws is more effective when accompanied by publicity aimed at:

— making people more alert to the risk of detection, arrest and its consequences;
— making drinking and driving less publicly acceptable;
— raising the acceptability of enforcement activities.

Public support for random breath testing, for instance, has remained high in New South Wales, Australia as a result of extensive public information concerning the measure.

A recent systematic review demonstrated that mass media campaigns that are carefully planned and well executed, that reach a sufficiently large audience, and that are implemented together with other prevention activities – such as highly-visible enforcement – are effective in reducing alcohol-impaired driving and alcohol-related crashes (*155*). In New Zealand, a recent evaluation of the five-year Supplementary Road Safety Package, which combines shock advertising with enforcement, found that this combination strategy saved between 285 and 516 lives over the five-year period (*156*).

Penalties for excess alcohol offenders

Prison sentences have been given for drink-driving offences in several countries, including Australia, Canada, Sweden and the United States. According to research, though, in the absence of effective enforcement such a penalty, in general, has been unsuccessful in deterring drinking drivers or reducing the rate of repeat offending (*148, 157*). If drivers perceive that the likelihood of their being detected and punished is low, then the effect of the penalty, even if severe, is likely to be small. All the same, research suggests that disqualification from driving after failing a breath test or refusing to take a breath test may deter drinking drivers – probably because of the swiftness and certainty of the punishment (*157*).

Interventions for high-risk offenders

High-risk offenders are usually defined as those with BAC levels in excess of 0.15 g/dl. In many industrialized countries, driver rehabilitation courses are available to offenders, though the components of such courses vary widely. Studies that have followed participants subsequent to drink-driving rehabilitation courses have shown, where participants are motivated to address their problems, that the courses reduce the rate of reoffending (*158, 159*).

Medicinal and recreational drugs

Legal requirements for police powers to carry out drug testing vary. Powers to carry out a blood or urine test exist in many countries to determine whether a driver is unfit to drive as a result of consuming drugs. The relationship between the use of drugs and involvement in road crashes is still largely unclear. Considerable research, though, is currently being undertaken to gain greater under-

standing of this subject. Enforcement strategies that deter people from driving while under the influence of drugs still have to be developed. Research is also being carried out in this area, to find efficient and cost-effective screening devices to help enforce laws on drug use and driving.

Drivers' hours of work in commercial and public transport

The previous chapter outlined the risks associated with cumulative fatigue as a result of lack of sleep, night driving and working shifts. Research indicates that fatigue is most prevalent among long-distance truck drivers (*160*) and that it is a factor in 20–30% of crashes in Europe and the United States involving commercial road vehicles (*161, 162*). A recent review of research on fatigue among commercial transport drivers in Australia found that between 10% and 50% of truck drivers drove while fatigued on a regular basis. The self-reported use of pills taken to stay awake in the long-distance road transport industry varies between 5% and 46% (*163*).

The normal pattern of work of commercial drivers is influenced by strong economic and social forces. Arguments about safety are usually ignored in many places, for commercial reasons (*161, 164–166*). However, an estimated 60% of the overall costs of traffic crashes involving commercial trucks in the United States are borne by society, rather than by the truck operators (*167*).

Working time – which often determines the time since the last significant period of sleep – is more critical to fatigue than actual driving time. Restrictions on driving hours that do not take into account when the driving occurs, forcing drivers to work according to shifting schedules, can result in greater sleep deprivation and make it difficult for the drivers' circadian rhythms to adapt (*161*).

Buses, coaches and commercial road transport are the only areas that are covered by specific legislation. It is increasingly recognized, though, that regulations on working and driving times need to be broadened. Drivers and operators, for instance, need training and information on fatigue and how to manage it. In Europe, in particular, laws on driving and working hours and their enforcement, over the last 30 years, have not yet reached the levels demanded by safety research (*161*). Safety experts believe that the policies on driving and working hour limits should take greater account of the scientific evidence on fatigue and crash risk and, in particular, of the following:

- *Daily and weekly rest.* The risk of being involved in a crash doubles after 11 hours of work (*168*). Sufficient time and proper facilities for meal breaks and daily rest and recuperation need to be provided. Where breaks cannot be taken at physiologically suitable times of the day, proper time must be given for full recuperation on a weekly, or shorter, basis.
- *Night work.* The risk of fatigue-related crashes at night is 10 times greater than during the day (*161*). The number of permissible working hours during the period of low circadian activity should be substantially less than the number permitted during the day.
- *Working and driving time.* There should be a coordinated approach to regulating driving and working time to ensure that permissible driving times do not inevitably lead to unacceptably high working times that double crash risk.

Some new vehicle technologies – such as on-board driver monitoring systems – promise to help in the detection of fatigue and excessive working hours. Road design standards urgently need to take better account of current knowledge of the causes and characteristics of crashes due to fatigue and inattention, and more research is needed to set good standards of road design to help prevent such crashes (*163*). While such technological advances can certainly help, none of them is a substitute for a proper regime of regulated working hours and its rigorous enforcement.

Cameras at traffic lights

Crashes at junctions are a leading source of road traffic injury. In addition to improved junction layout and design and the replacement, where appropriate, of signal-controlled junctions by roundabouts, research has shown that cameras can also be cost-effective in reducing crashes at junctions with traffic lights.

Cameras at traffic lights take photographs of vehicles going through the lights when the signal is red. In Australia, the introduction of such cameras in the late 1980s led to a 7% reduction in all crashes and a 32% reduction in front-to-side impacts at sites with cameras (*169*). In the United States, it was found that following the introduction of cameras at sites in Oxnard, California, the number of injury crashes fell by 29% and the number of front-to-side impacts involving injury fell by 68%, with no increase in rear impacts (*170*). A meta-analysis of studies of the effectiveness of cameras at traffic lights has shown that they are associated with a 12% reduction in the number of injury crashes (*16*). A cost–benefit analysis of cameras at traffic lights in the United Kingdom calculated that the return was nearly twice the investment after one year and 12 times the investment after five years (*171*).

Setting and enforcing seat-belt and child restraint use

Seat-belts

The level of seat-belt use is influenced by:

— whether there is legislation mandating their use;
— the degree to which enforcement of the law, complemented by publicity campaigns, is carried out;
— incentives offered to encourage use.

The time series shown in Figure is 4.1 is based on 30 years of experience in Finland with using seat-belts. It shows how legislation for compulsory use, without accompanying penalties, publicity or enforcement, has only a temporary effect on usage rates.

Mandatory seat-belt use laws

Mandatory seat-belt use has been one of road injury prevention's greatest success stories and has saved many lives. Occupant restraints first began to be fitted in cars in the late 1960s, and the first law on their mandatory use was passed in Victoria, Australia, in 1971. By the end of that year, the annual number of car occupant deaths in Victoria had fallen by 18%, and by 1975 by 26% (*173*). Following the experience of Victoria, many countries also introduced seat-belt laws, which have led to many hundreds of thousands of lives saved worldwide.

FIGURE 4.1

Use of seat-belts by car drivers/front-seat passengers in urban and non-urban areas of Finland, 1966–1995

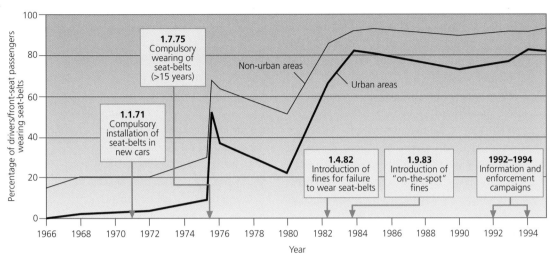

Source: reference *172.*

Seat-belts had been available for 20 years in Europe before their use was enforced by law, often with dramatic results. In the United Kingdom, for instance, front seat-belt usage rose from 37% before the introduction of the law to 95% a short period afterwards, with an accompanying fall of 35% in hospital admissions for road traffic injuries (*174, 175*). The wide variation in seat-belt use in European Union countries means that substantial further savings – estimated at around 7000 deaths annually – could be achieved if the usage rate was raised to the best that exists globally. In 1999, the best rates for seat-belt use recorded in high-income countries were in the 90–99% range for front-seat occupants, and in the 80–89% range for those in rear seats (*128*). Seat-belt use legislation in low-income countries is still not universal, and will become increasingly important as levels of car traffic rise.

The cost–benefit ratio of mandatory seat-belt use has been estimated at between 1:3 and 1:8 (*16*).

Enforcement and publicity

Research has shown that *primary enforcement* – where a driver is stopped solely for not wearing a seat-belt – is more effective than *secondary enforcement* – where a driver can only be stopped if another offence has been committed (*176, 177*). Primary enforcement

can increase seat-belt use, even where the level of use is already high (*178*).

Many studies, at both national and local levels, have shown that enforcement increases seat-belt use if it meets certain conditions. The enforcement needs to be selective, highly visible and well publicized, conducted over a sufficiently long period and repeated several times during a year (*179–183*). Selective Traffic Enforcement Programmes and similar programmes have been introduced in France, in parts of the Netherlands and in several states of the United States. Generally, wearing rates have been found to be around 10–15% higher than the baseline level, a year after the activities were carried out (*184*). Studies have estimated that the cost–benefit ratio of such seat-belt enforcement programmes is of the order of 1:3 or more (*172*).

The Selective Traffic Enforcement Programmes carried out in Canadian provinces have achieved improvements in seat-belt use, resulting in high rates of use. While the programmes differ across provinces in their details, their basic elements are broadly similar and include:

— an information briefing, educating police forces about the issue and its importance;

— following this campaign, a period of one to four weeks of intensive enforcement by the police, including fines, repeated several times a year;

— extensive public information and advertising;

— support for the enforcement campaigns in the media, and regular feedback in the media to public and police, on the progress recorded.

In the province of Saskatchewan, the programme has been repeated every year since 1988. In 1987, prior to the start of the programme seat-belt use of drivers was 72%, and that of front-seat passengers 67%. Figure 4.2 shows the incremental increases in seat-belt use – up to rates in excess of 90% – of drivers and front-seat passengers, from the introduction of the programme until 1994 (*185, 186*).

The reasons why this type of programme has had such success include (*186*):

• The programme is seen as a safety, rather than as an enforcement measure, as a result of public information before the programme started.

• The perceived risk of being caught is increased, because of the wide media coverage and police visibility.

• The provision of incentives (see below) strengthens the safety message and results in even higher police visibility.

• Feedback on the programme's progress motivates both the public and police.

• The programme is greater than the sum of its separate elements, that is to say, its individual elements reinforce each other.

In the Republic of Korea, in the second half of 2000, the government set a target to increase seat-belt use from 23% to 80% by 2006. By August 2001, efforts to increase seat-belt use that included publicity, enforcement and a 100% increase in fines for offenders, led to a spectacular increase in usage from 23% to 98%, a rate that was sustained in 2002 (*133*).

Six months after the introduction of legislation on seat-belt use in Thailand, a study in four cities found that the proportion of drivers wearing seat-belts had actually decreased. The reason for this is unclear, but it may have been related to problems with the consistent enforcement of the law (*187*).

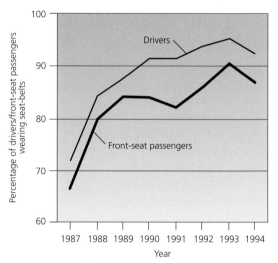

FIGURE 4.2

Use of seat-belts by car drivers/front-seat passengers in Saskatchewan, Canada, 1987–1994

Source: reference *185*.

Incentive programmes

Incentives programmes have been devised to enhance police enforcement of seat-belt use in a number of countries. In these programmes, seat-belt use is monitored and seat-belt wearers are eligible for a reward. The rewards may range from a meal voucher or lottery ticket to sizeable prizes such as video recorders or free holidays (*188*). In general, such programmes appear very effective and have a high level of acceptance. A meta-analysis of 34 studies examined the effects of incentives on seat-belt use, and found the size of the effect to be related to a number of variables, such as the target population, the initial baseline rate of seat-belt use and the prospect of immediate rewards (*184*).

Child restraints

The high level of effectiveness of child restraints in reducing fatal and serious injuries was discussed in the previous chapter. Good protection requires that the type of restraint used is appropriate for the age and weight of the child. Several restraint types exist and are covered by international standards. These include (*189*):

• *Rear-facing infant seats*: for infants up to 10 kg, from birth to 6–9 months, or for infants up to 13 kg, from birth to 12–15 months.

- *Forward-facing child seats*: for children weighing 9–18 kg, from approximately 9 months to 4 years.
- *Booster seats*: for children weighing 15–25 kg, aged from about 4 to 6 years.
- *Booster cushions*: for children weighing 22–36 kg, aged from about 6 to 11 years.

Effective interventions for increasing child restraint use include (*172, 190*):

— laws mandating child restraints;
— public information and enhanced enforcement campaigns;
— incentive programmes and education programmes to support enforcement;
— child restraint loan schemes.

In North America, children under 12 years are encouraged to sit in the rear of the vehicle, whereas in Europe, rear-facing child seats are increasingly being used on the front passenger seat. As mentioned in the previous chapter, while research has shown that rear-facing seats offer more protection than forward-facing seats, there are risks attached to placing rear-facing seats on the front seat directly in front of the passenger air bag. There should be clear instructions to avoid fitting rear-facing child restraints in this way. Devices exist that can automatically detect child restraints and occupants out of their normal position on the front seat, and switch off the passenger air bag.

As regards child restraint usage in low-income countries, cost and availability are important factors.

Mandatory child restraint laws

A review of studies on the effects of mandatory child restraint laws in the United States concluded that such laws have led to an average reduction of 35% in fatal injuries, a 17% decrease in all injuries and a 13% increase in child restraint use (*190, 191*).

While most cars in high-income countries are fitted with adult restraint systems, child restraint use requires informed decisions on the part of parents or guardians regarding design, availability and correct fitting. A further issue is the fact that age-related child seats can only be used for a limited period and the cost of replacing them could deter parents from doing so.

As mentioned earlier, the incorrect fitting and use of child equipment is a significant problem that decreases the potential safety benefits of these systems. Standardized anchorage points in cars would help to resolve many of these problems. Proposals for an international requirement have been discussed for many years, but not agreed as yet.

In the absence of child seats, it is important that adults are made to understand that they should avoid carrying children on their laps. The forces in a crash are such that, whatever action adults may take, they are unlikely to save an unbelted child from injury (*192*).

Child restraint loan programmes

Child restraint loan programmes are widely available in high-income countries. For a small fee or without charge, parents can have the loan of an infant seat from the maternity ward where the child is born. A further benefit of such schemes is their strong educational value and the opportunity they afford for precise advice to be given to the parents. The schemes have strongly affected usage rates of infant seats and also the use of appropriate child restraints throughout childhood (*191, 193*).

Setting and enforcing mandatory crash helmet use

Bicycle helmets

As already mentioned, the use of bicycle helmets has been found to reduce the risk of head and brain injuries by between 63% and 88% (*194–196*). As with other safety equipment, measures to increase the use of bicycle helmets involve a variety of strategies. A range of bicycle helmet standards is used worldwide. While there continues to be debate about whether mandatory use is appropriate – reflecting concerns that mandatory use could deter people from the otherwise healthy pursuit of cycling – the effectiveness of bicycle helmets for road safety is not at all in doubt (*195*) (see Box 4.5). In general, bicycle helmet use worldwide is low.

A meta-analysis of studies has shown that the mandatory wearing of cycle helmets has reduced the number of head injuries among cyclists by around 25% (*16*). In 1990, following 10 years of campaigns promoting the use of cycle helmets, the state of Victoria in Australia introduced the world's first law requiring cyclists to wear helmets. The rate of helmet wearing increased from 31% immediately before to 75% in the year following the new legislation and was associated with a 51% reduction in the numbers of crash victims who were admitted to hospital with head injuries or who died. Substantial increases in use were observed among all age groups, although rates of use were lowest among teenagers (*205*). Mandatory bicycle helmet laws introduced in New Zealand in 1994 also resulted in large increases in helmet use, and reductions in the number of head injuries of between 24% and 32% in non-motorized vehicle crashes and of 19% in motor vehicle crashes (*203*). Currently the rate of helmet wearing in New Zealand is around 90%, in all age groups (*206*).

Together with legislation on their use, helmet promotion programmes organized by community-wide groups, using a variety of educational and publicity strategies, have been shown to be effective in increasing helmet wearing in the United States (*207*). A law in Florida, United States, requires all riders under 16 years to wear a helmet; its introduction, which was accompanied by supporting strategies such as programmes in school on bicycle safety and the provision of free helmets for poorer people, led to a decline in the rate of bicycle-related injuries, from 73.3 to 41.8 per 100 000 population (*208*). In Canada, rates of helmet use rose rapidly following the introduction of mandatory laws for cyclists, and these rates were sustained over the next two years with regular education and enforcement by the police (*198*).

Cost–benefit ratios for cycle helmets have been estimated at around 1:6.2 for children, 1:3.3 for young adults and 1:2.7 for adults (*16*).

Motorcycle helmets

There are various strategies that effectively address the problem of head injuries in motorcyclists. They

---

BOX 4.5

Bicycle helmets

The incidence of bicycle-related injuries varies between countries. This is partly due to factors such as the road design, the traffic mix, climate and cultural attitudes (*197*). Over three quarters of fatal bicycle injuries are due to head injury (*198*). Among children, bicycle injuries are the leading cause of head injury (*199*).

There is now good evidence that bicycle helmets are effective in reducing head injuries. Early population-based research found that bicycle helmets reduced the risk of this type of injury by about 85% (*200*). More recent studies agree with this finding, with the estimated protective effects ranging from 47% to 88% (*195, 201*).

To promote the wearing of bicycle helmets, many governments have introduced legislation making bicycle helmets mandatory. During the 1990s, Australia, Canada, New Zealand and the United States brought in such laws. Since then, the Czech Republic, Finland, Iceland and Spain have followed suit. In the majority of cases, the laws have been directed at children and young people up to 18 years of age; only in Australia and New Zealand does the legislation cover bicyclists of all ages (*197*).

Evaluations of mandatory bicycle helmet laws have been encouraging. Findings from Canada, for instance, in those provinces where legislation has been introduced, show a 45% reduction in the rates of bicycle-related head injury (*202*). In New Zealand, it has been estimated that there was a 19% reduction in head injuries among cyclists over the first three years, following the introduction of bicycle helmet laws (*203*).

Those opposed to bicycle helmet legislation argue that wearing bicycle helmets encourages cyclists to take greater risks and therefore makes them more likely to incur injuries. To date, this argument has not found empirical evidence to support it. Other opponents have suggested that bicycle helmet legislation reduces the number of cyclists and it is for this reason that there are fewer head injuries. The most recent evidence, though, suggests the contrary: the number of child cyclists in Canada actually increased in the three years following the introduction of bicycle helmet laws (*204*).

There is unequivocal evidence that bicycle helmets reduce both the incidence and severity of head, brain and upper facial injuries. Making the wearing of bicycle helmets compulsory, together with improvements to the road environment that improve safety for cyclists, is therefore an effective strategy for reducing bicycle-related injuries.

include the introduction of performance standards for motorcycle safety helmets, legislation making helmet wearing compulsory – with penalties for non-use – and targeted information and enforcement campaigns.

In many parts of the world, helmet standards set out performance requirements for crash helmets. These standards are most effective when based on research findings on crash injury. A recent European initiative has recently reviewed, and subsequently revised, existing helmet standards in the light of current knowledge and crash research (*209*).

In low-income countries, it would be highly desirable for effective, comfortable and low-cost helmets to be developed and local manufacturing capacity increased. The Asia Injury Prevention Foundation, for instance, has developed a lightweight tropical helmet for use in Viet Nam and has drawn up standards for helmet performance. In Malaysia, the first standard for motorcycle helmets for adults was drafted in 1969 and updated in 1996. The country is now developing helmets specially designed for children (*210*).

Mandatory laws on helmet wearing

Increasing helmet wearing through the legislation requiring their use is important, especially in low-income countries where motorized two-wheeler use is high and current levels of helmet wearing low. It has been suggested that when a motorcycle is purchased, the acquisition of an approved helmet should be mandated, or at least encouraged, especially in low-income countries (*17*).

In Malaysia, where legislation on the use of helmets was introduced in 1973, it was estimated that the law led to a reduction of about 30% in motorcycle deaths (*211*). In Thailand, in the year following the enforcement of the law on wearing helmets, their use increased five-fold, while motorcycle head injuries decreased by 41.4% and deaths by 20.8% (*212*).

An evaluation of helmet use and traumatic brain injury, before and after the introduction of legislation, in the region of Romagna, Italy, found that helmet use increased from an average of less than 20% in 1999 to over 96% in 2001, and was

an effective measure for preventing traumatic brain injury at all ages (*213*).

A meta-analysis of studies – mainly from the United States, where many laws on helmets were introduced in the period 1967–1970, around a half of which were repealed between 1976 and 1978 – found that the introduction of laws on compulsory helmet wearing reduced the number of injuries to moped riders and motorcyclists by 20–30% (*16*). Similarly, the analysis of the effects of repealing helmet wearing laws showed that withdrawing them led to an increase of around 30% in the numbers of fatal injuries, and an increase of 5–10% in injuries to moped riders and motorcyclists (*16*). A recent study on the repeal of laws in the United States found that observed helmet use in the states of Kentucky and Louisiana dropped from nearly full compliance, when the laws were still operative, to around 50%. After the repeal of the laws, motorcycle deaths increased by 50% in Kentucky and by 100% in Louisiana (*214*).

Economic evaluations of mandatory helmet wearing laws, based largely on experience in the United States, found high cost–benefit ratios, ranging from 1:1.3 to 1:16 (*215*).

The role of education, information and publicity

Public health sector campaigns in the field of road injury prevention have encompassed a wide range of measures, but education has always featured as the mainstay of prevention (*216*). In the light of ongoing research and experience of the systems approach to road injury prevention, many professionals in the field have re-examined the role that education plays in prevention (*26, 216, 217*). It is clear that informing and educating road users can improve knowledge about the rules of the road and about such matters as purchasing safer vehicles and equipment. Basic skills on how to control vehicles can be taught. Education can help to bring about a climate of concern and develop sympathetic attitudes towards effective interventions. Consultation with road users and residents is essential in designing urban safety management schemes.

As the previous section showed, when used in support of legislation and law enforcement, publicity and information can create shared social norms for safety. However, when used in isolation, education, information and publicity do not generally deliver tangible and sustained reductions in deaths and serious injuries (*26, 190, 217*). Historically, considerable emphasis has been placed on efforts to reduce road user error through traffic safety education – for example, in pedestrian and cycle education for school children, and in advanced and remedial driver training schemes. Although such efforts can be effective in changing behaviour (*218*), there is no

evidence that they have been effective in reducing rates of road traffic crashes (*218, 219*) (see Box 4.6).

Delivering post-crash care
Chain of help for patients injured in road crashes

The aim of post-impact care is to avoid preventable death and disability, to limit the severity of the injury and the suffering caused by it, and to ensure the crash survivor's best possible recovery and reintegration into society. The way in which those

---

BOX 4.6

Educational approaches to pedestrian safety

Educating pedestrians on how to cope with the traffic environment is considered an essential component of strategies to reduce pedestrian injuries and has been recommended in all types of countries.

In order to reach the two groups of pedestrians that are particularly vulnerable – children and older people – educational programmes use a variety of methods, frequently in combination. These approaches include talks, printed materials, films, multi-media kits, table-top models, mock-ups of intersections, songs and other forms of music. Education is provided either directly to the target population or indirectly – through parents or teachers, for instance – and in various settings, such as the home, the classroom or a real traffic situation.

Most studies on the effectiveness of educational programmes report on surrogate outcomes, such as observed or reported behaviour, attitudes and knowledge. From a public health perspective, though, the main outcomes of interest are crashes, deaths, injuries and disabilities. The studies reporting these outcomes tend to have methodological limitations which reduce their usefulness for comparative purposes. Limitations include the absence of randomization for assigning subjects to intervention and control groups (*220–223*), the absence of detailed data for control groups (*221*), or the lack of a control group (*224*).

A systematic review (*218*), including 15 randomized controlled trials that measured the effectiveness of programmes of safety education for pedestrians, found:

- There was a lack of good evidence for adults, particularly in the case of elderly people.
- There was a lack of good evidence from low-income and middle-income countries.
- The quality of the studies was fairly poor, even in randomized controlled studies.
- The variety of intervention models and of methods of measuring outcomes made comparisons between studies difficult.
- Only surrogate outcomes were reported.
- While a change in knowledge and attitudes in children was confirmed, the size of the measured effect varied considerably.
- A change in behaviour was found in children, but not in all studies, and the size of the effect was influenced by the method of measuring, as well as by the context, such as whether a child was alone or with other children.
- The effect of education on the risk of a pedestrian incurring an injury remains uncertain.

Overall, the effect of safety education of pedestrians on behaviour varied considerably. Knowledge of pedestrian safety in children can translate into changed attitudes and even into appropriate forms of behaviour, but there is uncertainty about the extent to which the observed behavioural changes persist over time. There is no evidence that observed behaviour is causally related to the risk of occurrence of pedestrian injury. If it is, though, there is no reliable information about the size of the effect of pedestrian behaviour on the frequency of pedestrian injuries. Reliable scientific information on the effectiveness of educational approaches to pedestrian safety in low-income and middle-income countries is lacking. Also needing more research is the effectiveness of educational approaches in all countries with elderly pedestrians.

injured in road crashes are dealt with following a crash crucially determines their chances and the quality of survival.

A study in high-income countries found that about 50% of deaths from road traffic crashes occurred within minutes, either at the scene or while in transit to hospital. For those patients taken to hospital, around 15% of deaths occurred within the first four hours after the crash, but a much greater proportion, around 35%, occurred after four hours (*225*). In reality, therefore, there is not so much a "golden hour" in which interventions have to take place (*226*) as a chain of opportunities for intervening across a longer timescale. This chain involves bystanders at the scene of the crash, emergency rescue, access to the emergency care system, and trauma care and rehabilitation.

Pre-hospital care

As already pointed out in the previous chapter, the vast majority of road traffic deaths in low-income and middle-income countries occur in the pre-hospital phase (*227*). In Malaysia, for instance, 72% of motorcycle deaths occur during this phase (*228*). At least half of all trauma deaths in high-income countries are pre-hospital deaths (*225, 227*). A number of options exist for improving the quality of pre-hospital care. Even where these options are cheap, they are frequently not taken up to sufficient extent (*229*).

Role of lay bystanders

Those who are present or who arrive first at the scene of a crash can play an important role in various ways, including:

— contacting the emergency services, or calling for other forms of help;
— helping to put out any fire;
— taking action to secure the scene (e.g. preventing further crashes, preventing harm to rescuers and bystanders, controlling the crowd gathered at the scene);
— applying first aid.

Many deaths from airway obstruction or external haemorrhage could be avoided by lay bystanders trained in first aid (*230*).

In low-income and some middle-income countries, rescue by ambulance occurs in the minority of cases and assistance from a lay bystander is the main source of health care for the victims. In Ghana, for example, the majority of injured patients who reach hospital do so by means of some form of commercial vehicle (*227, 231*). It has been suggested that basic first-aid training for commercial drivers might be helpful (*227*), though it has not been scientifically established whether such a measure would decrease pre-hospital mortality (*229*).

A pilot project on pre-hospital care training was conducted in Cambodia and northern Iraq, in areas with a high density of landmines where people were frequently injured (*232*). The first stage of the project involved giving 5000 lay people a basic two-day training course in first aid. These people would be "first responders" in landmine explosions. In the second stage, paramedics were given 450 hours of formal training. A rigorous evaluation was conducted of the effects of the project on landmine-related injuries in the two areas, using an injury surveillance system. Among those severely injured in the areas covered by the project, the mortality rate fell from 40% before the project to 9% afterwards. The project relied on training and some basic supplies and equipment, but did not provide vehicles, such as formal ambulances. Transportation continued to be provided by the existing system of public and private vehicles in each area.

Similar pilot programmes have taken place, or are being conducted, involving training for lay "first responders" or others who are not health care professionals but who might have occasion to come upon injured people on a regular basis. They include training for police in Uganda and for the lay public generally in India, though evaluations have not yet been published of these two programmes.

Programmes providing first-aid training to the lay public, either generally or to particular population groups – such as the police, commercial drivers or village health workers – should follow certain principles to help strengthen their impact. For instance, such programmes should:

— base the contents of their training on epide-

miological patterns in the particular area in which they are to operate;
— standardize training internationally;
— monitor the results;
— plan periodic refresher courses, using results of monitoring to modify the contents of the training.

Access to the emergency medical system

In low-income countries, the development of the emergency medical system is limited by economic constraints and by the restricted availability of tele-communications. While some low-income countries have started rudimentary ambulance services in urban areas, they are still the exception as far as most of sub-Saharan Africa and southern Asia is concerned (*229*). International reviews have urged caution in transferring emergency medical systems from high-income countries to low-income countries, questioning whether such actions represent the best use of scarce resources. Another concern is the lack of conclusive evidence on the benefits of some Advanced Life Support measures commonly used in high-income areas, such as pre-hospital endotracheal intubation and intravenous fluid resuscitation (*233–235*). Further research is clearly needed on the effectiveness and cost-effectiveness of such more advanced measures. Research is equally called for on the role of Basic Life Support training in low-income countries – particularly in rural areas, where there is no formal emergency medical system and it might take days to reach professional medical care (*229*).

In high-income countries, access to the emergency medical system is almost always made by tele-phone, but the coverage and reliability of the telephone link varies between countries. The growth in the use of mobile telephones, even in low-income and middle-income countries, has radically improved emergency access to medical and other assistance. In many countries, there is a standard emergency telephone number that can be dialled for urgent assistance. Uniform codes for emergency assistance, for land telephones and mobile phones, should be set up in all regions of the world.

Emergency rescue services

Police and firefighters often arrive at the crash scene before personnel from the emergency medical service. Early intervention by firefighters and rescuers is critical where people are trapped in a vehicle, particularly if it is on fire or submerged under water. Firefighters and police need to be trained, therefore, in basic life support. There should be close cooperation between firefighters and other groups of rescuers, as well as between firefighters and health care providers (*225*).

As mentioned earlier, there are risks associated with ambulance transport, both for those transported by the ambulance as well as people in the street. Safety standards must therefore be established for transportation by ambulance – for instance, on the use of child restraints and adult seat-belts.

The hospital setting

There is growing understanding in high-income countries of the principal components of hospital trauma care and an awareness of what aspects require further research. Many improvements have taken place in trauma care over the last 30 years, largely as a result of new technology and improvements in organization (*236*). Clinical capabilities and staffing, equipment and supplies, and trauma care organization are all issues considered by medical experts to be of great importance (*225, 237*).

Human resources

Training for teams managing trauma care is vital. It is generally acknowledged that the standard for such training in high-income countries is the Advanced Trauma Life Support course of the American College of Surgeons (*225, 229, 238*). The applicability of this course to low-income and middle-income countries, though, has yet to be established.

The problems faced by low-income countries in relation to human resources, equipment and the organization of services have already been discussed. Though little has been documented on effective ways to deal with these problems, there is some evidence of successful practice (*229*). In Trinidad and Tobago, for instance, the introduction of the Advanced Trauma Life Support course for doctors and the Pre-Hospital Trauma Life Support course for paramedics, together with improved emergency equipment, led to improvements in trauma care and a decrease in trauma mortality, both in the field and in hospital (*239*).

South Africa (a middle-income country) also runs Advanced Trauma Life Support courses for doctors (*240*), though a cost–benefit analysis of this training has not been performed. Several low-income countries in Africa have adapted South Africa's programme to their own circumstances, which generally include a lack of high-tech equipment and practical difficulties in referring patients to higher levels of care (*236*).

Apart from short in-service training, there also needs to be more formal, in-depth training. This includes improving the trauma-related training received by doctors, nurses and other professionals, both in their basic education and in postgraduate training.

Physical resources

Many hospitals in low-income and middle-income countries lack important trauma-related equipment, some of which is not expensive.

In Ghana, for instance, as mentioned in the previous chapter, a survey of 11 rural hospitals found that none had chest tubes and only four had emergency airway equipment. Such equipment is vital for treating life-threatening chest injuries and airway obstruction, major preventable causes of death in trauma patients. All of it is cheap and much is reusable. The survey suggested that a lack of organization and planning, rather than restricted resources, was to blame (*241*). Similar deficiencies have been documented in other countries. In public hospitals in Kenya, shortages of oxygen, blood for transfusion, antiseptics, anaesthetics and intravenous fluids have been recorded (*242*). Research is urgently needed on this problem. It is important, too, to draw on relevant experience from other fields. National blood transfusion centres, for example, with their management of blood for transfusions – which involves recruiting suitable donors and collecting blood, screening donated blood for transfusion-transmissible infections, and ensuring that a safe blood supply is constantly available at places throughout the country.

Organization of trauma care

A prerequisite for high-quality trauma care in hospital emergency departments is the existence of a strategy for the planning, organization and provision of a national trauma system. There is considerable potential worldwide to upgrade arrangements for trauma care and improve training in trauma care at the primary health care level, in district hospitals and in tertiary care hospitals. International guidelines for this, based on research, need to be established.

The Essential Trauma Care Project is a collaborative effort between the WHO and the International Society of Surgery that aims to improve the planning and organization of trauma care worldwide (*243*). The project seeks to help individual counties, in developing their own trauma services, to:

— define a core of essential injury treatment services;

— define the human and physical resources necessary to assure such services in the best possible way, given particular economic and geographic contexts;

— develop administrative mechanisms to promote these and related resources on a national and international basis; such mechanisms will include specific training programmes, programmes to improve quality and hospital inspections.

While the goals of the Essential Trauma Care Project extend beyond the field of road safety, the success of the project can only be beneficial for crash-related trauma care.

Rehabilitation

For every person who dies in a road traffic crash, many more are left with permanent disabilities.

Rehabilitation services are an essential component of the comprehensive package of initial and post-hospital care of the injured. They help to minimize future functional disabilities and restore the injured person to an active life within society. The importance of early rehabilitation has been proved, though best practice in treatment programmes has yet to be identified (*225*). Most countries need to increase the capacity of their health care systems to provide adequate rehabilitation to survivors of road traffic crashes.

High-quality treatment and interventions for rehabilitation during the period of hospitalization immediately following an injury are of utmost importance, in order to prevent life-threatening complications related to immobilization. However, despite the best management, many people will still become disabled as a consequence of road traffic crashes. In low-income and middle-income countries, efforts should focus on capacity building and personnel training so as to improve the management of survivors of road traffic crashes in the acute phase, and thus prevent, as far as possible, the development of permanent disability.

Medical rehabilitation services involve professionals from a range of disciplines. These include specialists in physical medicine and rehabilitation, as well as in other medical or paramedical fields, such as orthopaedics, neurosurgery and general surgery, physical and occupational therapy, prosthetics and orthotics, psychology, neuropsychology, speech pathology and nursing. In every case, the recovery of both the patient's physical and mental health is paramount, as well as their ability to become independent again and participate in daily life.

Medical rehabilitation services also play a vital part in helping those living with disabilities to achieve independence and a good quality of life. Among other things, these services can provide mechanical aids that greatly assist affected individuals to be reintegrated into, and participate in, ordinary daily activities, including their work. Such aids, delivered through outpatient departments or outreach services to the home, are often essential in preventing further deterioration. In many countries, once acute management has been accomplished and mechanical aids provided, community-based rehabilitation remains the only realistic means of reintegrating the individual into society.

Research

Much of the research on the effectiveness and cost–benefits of interventions takes place in high-income countries. The development of national research capacity is thus an urgent need in many other parts of the world (*244, 245*). Experience from high-income countries shows the importance of having at least one – preferably independent – national organization receiving solid core funding that deals with road safety research.

Encouraging the development of professional expertise across a range of disciplines at national level, together with regional cooperation and exchange of information, have reaped much benefit in industrialized countries. Developing these mechanisms should be a priority where they do not exist. Among the many research-related needs for road injury prevention, the following are some of the more pressing:

- Better collection and analysis of data, so as to enable more reliable estimates to be made of the global burden of road traffic injuries, especially in low-income and middle-income countries. This includes mortality data, conforming to internationally-standardized definitions, and data on acute morbidity and long-term disability. There should also be more research to find low-cost methods of obtaining these data.
- Further data on the economic and social impacts of road traffic injuries, especially in low-income and middle-income countries. There is a considerable lack of economic analysis in the field of road injury prevention in these countries. The cost of injuries is not known empirically, neither are the cost nor cost-effectiveness of interventions.
- Studies demonstrating the effectiveness of specific interventions for injuries in low-income and middle-income countries.
- Design standards and guidelines for intercity roads carrying mixed traffic.

The following areas require particular research:
— how best to assess the effectiveness of packages of road safety measures combining different actions, such as area-wide traffic calming and urban design;
— the interaction between transport planning and urban and regional planning, and how these affect road safety;
— the design of roads and traffic management, taking into account traffic environments and

traffic mixes encountered in low-income and middle-income countries;

— how successfully various types of preventive measures can be transferred between countries with differing socioeconomic conditions and differing rates of motorization and traffic mixes.

Research in low-income and middle-income countries needs to be carried out on a regional basis towards developing the following:

— light, well-ventilated motorcycle helmets;
— safer bus and truck fronts;
— standards for motorcycle crash protection;
— the visibility and crash protection of indigenously-designed vehicles.

Improvements in post-impact care at an affordable cost are a priority area for the health sector. Equally important is research to better understand the mechanisms causing head injury and whiplash injury in road crashes, and treatments for these injuries. There is currently, for instance, no effective pharmacological treatment for head injury.

In all countries, further research is required into managing exposure to risk – the least-used injury prevention strategy. It is also essential to resolve the growing incompatibility in many places between smaller, lighter vehicles and larger, heavier ones.

Conclusion

Substantial research and development over the last 30 years have proved that a range of interventions exist to prevent road crashes and injury. The gap, though, between what is known to be effective and what is actually practised is often considerable. As with other areas of public health, road injury prevention requires effective management to put in place sustainable, evidence-based measures, overcoming obstacles to their implementation.

Good transport and land-use policies offer a means of reducing the exposure to risk for road crash injury. Safety-conscious planning and design of the road network can minimize the risk of crashes and crash injury. Crash-protective features on a vehicle can save lives and reduce injuries for road users, both inside and outside the vehicle. Compliance with key road safety rules can be signifi-

cantly increased using a combination of legislation, enforcement of the laws, and information and education. The availability of good quality emergency care can save lives, and greatly reduce the severity and long-term consequences of road injuries.

A large proportion of road traffic injuries in low-income and middle-income countries occur among vulnerable road users. An important priority must therefore be to introduce a wide range of measures that give these road users greater protection. All the prevention strategies described in this report call for a wide mobilization of effort, at all levels, involving close collaboration across many disciplines and sectors, prominent among which is the health sector.

Despite many attempts to find and document examples of "good practice" in road safety in developing countries, such examples seem to be few. This chapter, therefore, remains slanted to a description of what has been successful in highly-motorized countries. This is not to say that the interventions presented in this chapter will not work in low-income or middle-income countries – indeed, many of them do. There needs, though, to be further testing of prevention strategies, to find ways to adapt them to local conditions – and not merely to adopt and apply them unchanged.

References

1. Bolen J et al. Overview of efforts to prevent motor vehicle-related injury. In: Bolen J, Sleet DA, Johnson V, eds. *Prevention of motor vehicle-related injuries: a compendium of articles from the Morbidity and Mortality Weekly Report, 1985–1996*. Atlanta, GA, Centers for Disease Control and Prevention, 1997.

2. Dora C, Phillips M, eds. *Transport, environment and health*. Copenhagen, World Health Organization Regional Office for Europe, 2000 (European Series No. 89)(http://www.who.dk/document/e72015.pdf, accessed 17 November 2003).

3. Evans L. The new traffic safety vision for the United States. *American Journal of Public Health*, 2003, 93:1384–1386.

4. Koornstra M et al. *Sunflower: a comparative study of the development of road safety in Sweden, the United Kingdom and the Netherlands*. Leidschendam, Institute for Road Safety Research, 2002.

5. Rumar K. *Transport safety visions, targets and strategies: beyond 2000.* Brussels, European Transport Safety Council, 1999 (1st European Transport Safety Lecture) (http://www.etsc.be/eve.htm, accessed 30 October 2003).

6. Litman T. *If health matters: integrating public health objectives in transportation planning.* Victoria, BC, Victoria Transport Policy Institute, 2003 (http://www.vtpi.org/health.pdf, accessed 4 December 2003).

7. Rodriguez DY, Fernandez FJ, Velasquez HA. Road traffic injuries in Colombia. *Injury Control and Safety Promotion*, 2003, 10:29–35.

8. *TransMilenio. A high capacity/low cost bus rapid transit system developed for Bogotá, Colombia.* Bogotá, Trans-Milenio SA, 2001.

9. Hummel T. *Land use planning in safer transportation network planning.* Leidschendam, Institute for Road Safety Research, 2001 (SWOV Report D-2001-12).

10. Ross A et al., eds. *Towards safer roads in developing countries. A guide for planners and engineers.* Crowthorne, Transport Research Laboratory, 1991.

11. Aeron-Thomas A et al. *A review of road safety management and practice. Final report.* Crowthorne, Transport Research Laboratory and Babtie Ross Silcock, 2002 (TRL Report PR/INT216/2002).

12. Allsop R. *Road safety audit and safety impact assessment.* Brussels, European Transport Safety Council, 1997.

13. Wegman FCM et al. *Road safety impact assessment.* Leidschendam, Institute for Road Safety Research, 1994 (SWOV Report R-94-20).

14. Hummel T. *Route management in safer transportation network planning.* Leidschendam, Institute for Road Safety Research, 2001 (SWOV Report D-2001-11).

15. Allsop RE, ed. *Safety of pedestrians and cyclists in urban areas.* Brussels, European Transport Safety Council, 1999 (http://www.etsc.be/rep.htm, accessed 17 November 2003).

16. Elvik R, Vaa T. *Handbook of road safety measures.* Amsterdam, Elsevier, in press.

17. Forjuoh SN. Traffic-related injury prevention interventions for low income countries. *Injury Control and Safety Promotion*, 2003, 10:109–118.

18. Hijar M, Vasquez-Vela E, Arreola-Rissa C. Pedestrian traffic injuries in Mexico. *Injury Control and Safety Promotion*, 2003, 10:37–43.

19. Mutto M, Kobusingye OC, Lett RR. The effect of an overpass on pedestrian injuries on a major highway in Kampala, Uganda. *African Health Science*, 2002, 2:89–93.

20. Litman T. *Distance-based vehicle insurance: feasibility, costs and benefits. Comprehensive Technical Report.* Victoria, BC, Victoria Transport Policy Institute, 2000 (http://www.vtpi.org/dbvi_com.pdf, accessed 5 December 2003).

21. Edlin AS. *Per-mile premiums for auto insurance.* Berkeley, CA, Department of Economics, University of California, 2002 (Working Paper E02-318) (http://repositories.cdlib.org/iber/econ/E02-318, accessed 5 December 2003).

22. *PROMISING. Promotion of mobility and safety of vulnerable road users.* Leidschendam, Institute for Road Safety Research, 2001.

23. Mohan D, Tiwari G. Road safety in low-income countries: issues and concerns regarding technology transfer from high-income countries. In: *Reflections on the transfer of traffic safety knowledge to motorising nations.* Melbourne, Global Traffic Safety Trust, 1998:27–56.

24. Mayhew DR, Simpson HM. *Motorcycle engine size and traffic safety.* Ottawa, Traffic Injury Research Foundation of Canada, 1989.

25. Broughton J. *The effect on motorcycling of the 1981 Transport Act.* Crowthorne, Transport and Road Research Laboratory, 1987 (Research Report No. 106).

26. Trinca GW et al. *Reducing traffic injury: the global challenge.* Melbourne, Royal Australasian College of Surgeons, 1988.

27. *Motorcycling safety position paper.* Birmingham, Royal Society for the Prevention of Accidents, 2001.

28. Norghani M et al. *Use of exposure control methods to tackle motorcycle accidents in Malaysia.* Serdang, Road Safety Research Centre, Universiti Putra Malaysia, 1998 (Research Report 3/98).

29. Williams AF. An assessment of graduated licensing legislation. In: *Proceedings of the 47th Association for the Advancement of Automotive Medicine (AAAM) conference, Lisbon, Portugal, 22–24 September 2003.* Washington, DC, Association for the

Advancement of Automotive Medicine, 2003: 533–535.

30. Waller P. The genesis of GDL. *Journal of Safety Research, 2003*, 34:17–23.

31. Williams AF, Ferguson SA. Rationale for graduated licensing and the risks it should address. *Injury Prevention*, 2002, 8:9–16.

32. *Graduated driver licensing model law, approved October 24, 1996, by NCUTLO membership (revised 1999, 2000)*. National Committee on Uniform Traffic Laws and Ordinances, 2000 (http://www.ncutlo.org/gradlaw2.html, accessed 11 December 2003).

33. *Licensing systems for young drivers, as of December 2003*. Insurance Institute for Highway Safety/Highway Loss Data Institute, 2003 (http://www.highwaysafety.org/safety_facts/state_laws/grad_license.htm, accessed 11 December 2003).

34. Shope JT, Molnar LJ. Graduated driver licensing in the United States: evaluation results from the early programs. *Journal of Safety Research*, 2003, 34:63–69.

35. Simpson HM. The evolution and effectiveness of graduated licensing. *Journal of Safety Research*, 2003, 34:25–34.

36. Begg D, Stephenson S. Graduated driver licensing: the New Zealand experience. *Journal of Safety Research*, 2003, 34:99–105.

37. Foss R, Goodwin A. Enhancing the effectiveness of graduated driver licensing legislation. *Journal of Safety Research*, 2003, 34:79–84.

38. Wegman F, Elsenaar P. *Sustainable solutions to improve road safety in the Netherlands*. Leidschendam, Institute for Road Safety Research, 1997 (SWOV Report D-097-8).

39. Ogden KW. *Safer roads: a guide to road safety engineering*. Melbourne, Ashgate Publishing Ltd, 1996.

40. *Cities on the move: a World Bank urban strategy review*. Washington, DC, The World Bank, 2002.

41. *Handboek: categorisering wegen op duurzaam veilige basis. Deel I (Voorlopige): functionele en operationele eisen [Handbook: categorizing roads on long-lasting safe basis. Part I (Provisional): functional and operational demands]*. Ede, Stichting centrum voor regelgeving en onderoek in de grond-, water- en wegenbouw en de verkeerstechniek, 1997 (CROW Report 116).

42. *Zone guide for pedestrian safety shows how to make systematic improvements*. Washington, DC, National Highway Traffic Safety Administration, 1998 (Technology Transfer Series Number 181) (http://www.nhtsa.dot.gov/people/outreach/traftech/pub/tt181.html, accessed 5 December 2003).

43. *Towards a sustainable safe traffic system in the Netherlands*. Leidschendam, Institute for Road Safety Research, 1993.

44. *Ville plus sûr, quartiers sans accidents: realisations; evaluations [Safer city, districts without accidents: achievements; evaluations]*. Lyon, Centre d'études sur les réseaux, les transports, l'urbanisme et les constructions publiques, 1994.

45. *Safety strategies for rural roads*. Paris, Organisation for Economic Co-operation and Development, 1999 (http://www.oecd.org/dataoecd/59/2/2351720.pdf, accessed 17 December 2003).

46. Afukaar FK, Antwi P, Ofosu-Amah S. Pattern of road traffic injuries in Ghana: implications for control. *Injury Control and Safety Promotion*, 2003, 10:69–76.

47. *Safety of vulnerable road users*. Paris, Organisation for Economic Co-operation and Development, 1998 (DSTI/DOT/RTR/RS7(98)1/FINAL) (http://www.oecd.org/dataoecd/24/4/2103492.pdf, accessed 17 November 2003).

48. Ossenbruggen PJ, Pendharkar J, Ivan J. Roadway safety in rural and small urbanized areas. *Accident Analysis and Prevention*, 2001, 33:485–498.

49. Khan FM et al. Pedestrian environment and behavior in Karachi, Pakistan. *Accident Analysis and Prevention*, 1999, 31:335–339.

50. Herrstedt L. Planning and safety of bicycles in urban areas. In: *Proceedings of the Traffic Safety on Two Continents Conference, Lisbon, 22–24 September 1997*. Linköping, Swedish National Road and Transport Research Institute, 1997:43–58.

51. Kjemtrup K, Herrstedt L. Speed management and traffic calming in urban areas in Europe: a historical view. *Accident Analysis and Prevention*, 1992, 24:57–65.

52. Brilon W, Blanke H. Extensive traffic calming: results of the accident analyses in six model towns. In: *ITE 1993 Compendium of Technical Papers*. Washington, DC, Institute of Transportation Engineers, 1993:119–123.

53. Herrstedt L et al. *An improved traffic environment.* Copenhagen, Danish Road Directorate, 1993 (Report No. 106).

54. *Guidelines for urban safety management.* London, Institution of Highways and Transportation, 1990.

55. Lines CJ, Machata K. Changing streets, protecting people: making roads safer for all. In: *Proceedings of the Best in Europe Conference, Brussels, 12 September 2000.* Brussels, European Transport Safety Council, 2000:37–47.

56. Elvik R. *Cost-benefit analysis of safety measures for vulnerable and inexperienced road users.* Oslo, Institute of Transport Economics, 1999 (EU Project PROMISING, TØI Report 435/1999).

57. Bunn F et al. Traffic calming for the prevention of road traffic injuries: systematic review and meta-analysis. *Injury Prevention*, 2003, 9: 200–204.

58. *Guidelines for the safety audit of roads and road project in Malaysia.* Kuala Lumpur, Roads Branch, Public Works Department, 1997.

59. *Guidelines for road safety audit.* London, Institution of Highways and Transportation, 1996.

60. *Road safety audit*, 2nd ed. Sydney, Austroads, 2002.

61. Macaulay J, McInerney R. *Evaluation of the proposed actions emanating from road safety audits.* Sydney, Austroads, 2002 (Austroads Publication No. AP-R209/02).

62. *Accident countermeasures: literature review.* Wellington, Transit New Zealand, 1992 (Research Report No. 10).

63. Schelling A. Road safety audit, the Danish experience. In: *Proceedings of the Forum of European Road Safety Research Institutes (FERSI) International Conference on Road Safety in Europe and Strategic Highway Research Program, Prague, September 1995.* Linköping, Swedish National Road and Transport Research Institute, 1995:1–8.

64. *Roadside obstacles.* Paris, Organisation for Economic Co-operation and Development, 1975.

65. *Forgiving roadsides.* Brussels, European Transport Safety Council, 1998 (http://www.etsc.be/bri_road5.pdf, accessed 10 December 2003).

66. Cirillo JA, Council FM. Highway safety: twenty years later. *Transportation Research Record*, 1986, 1068:90–95.

67. Ross HE et al. *Recommended procedures for the safety performance evaluation of highway features.* Washington, DC, National Co-operative Highway Research Program, 1993 (Report No. 350).

68. Carlsson A, Brüde U. *Utvärdering av mötesfri väg [Evaluation of roads designed to prevent head-on crashes].* Linköping, Swedish National Road and Transport Research Institute, 2003 (VTI Report No. 45-2003) (http://www.vti.se/PDF/reports/N45-2003.pdf, accessed 10 December 2003).

69. *Research on loss of control accidents on Warwickshire motorways and dual carriageways.* Coventry, TMS Consultancy, 1994.

70. Elvik R, Rydningen U. *Effektkatalog for trafikksikkerhetstiltak. [A catalogue of estimates of effects of road safety measures].* Oslo, Institute of Transport Economics, 2002, (TØI Report 572/2002) (http://www.toi.no/toi_Data/Attachments/909/r572_02.pdf, accessed 17 December 2003).

71. Allsop RE, ed. *Low cost road and traffic engineering measures for casualty reduction.* Brussels, European Transport Safety Council, 1996.

72. Koornstra M, Bijleveld F, Hagenzieker M. *The safety effects of daytime running lights.* Leidschendam, Institute for Road Safety Research, 1997 (SWOV Report R-97-36).

73. Farmer CM, Williams AF. Effect of daytime running lights on multiple vehicle daylight crashes in the United States. *Accident Analysis and Prevention*, 2002, 34:197–203.

74. Hollo P. Changes in the legislation on the use of daytime running lights by motor vehicles and their effect on road safety in Hungary. *Accident Analysis and Prevention*, 1998, 30:183–199.

75. *Cost-effective EU transport safety measures.* Brussels, European Transport and Safety Council, 2003 (http://www.etsc.be/costeff.pdf, accessed 10 December 2003).

76. Zador PL. Motorcycle headlight-use laws and fatal motorcycle crashes in the US, 1975–1983. *American Journal of Public Health*, 1985, 75:543–546.

77. Yuan W. The effectiveness of the "ride bright" legislation for motorcycles in Singapore. *Accident Analysis and Prevention*, 2000, 32:559–563.

78. Radin Umar RS, Mackay MG, Hills BL. Modelling of conspicuity-related motorcycle acci-

dents in Seremban and Shah Alam, Malaysia. *Accident Analysis and Prevention*, 1996, 28:325–332.

79. Mohan D, Patel R. Development and promotion of a safety shopping bag vest in developing countries. *Applied Ergonomics*, 1990, 21:346–347.

80. Kwan I, Mapstone J. Interventions for increasing pedestrian and cyclist visibility for the prevention of death and injuries. *Cochrane Database of Systematic Reviews*, 2002, (2):CD003438.

81. *NHTSA vehicle safety rulemaking priorities and supporting research, 2003–2006.* Washington, DC, National Highway Traffic Safety Administration, 2003 (Docket No. NHTSA-2003-15505)(http://www.nhtsa.dot.gov/cars/rules/rulings/PriorityPlan/FinalVeh/Index.html, accessed 10 December 2003).

82. Mackay GM, Wodzin E. Global priorities for vehicle safety. In: *International Conference on Vehicle Safety 2002: IMechE conference transactions.* London, Institution of Mechanical Engineers, 2002:3–9.

83. *Priorities for EU motor vehicle safety design.* Brussels, European Transport Safety Council, Vehicle Safety Working Party, 2001.

84. Broughton J et al. *The numerical context for setting national casualty reduction targets.* Crowthorne, Transport Research Laboratory Ltd, 2000 (TRL Report No. 382).

85. *Road safety strategy 2010.* Wellington, National Road Safety Committee, Land Transport Safety Authority, 2000.

86. *Reducing traffic injuries through vehicle safety improvements: the role of car design.* Brussels, European Transport Safety Council, 1993.

87. *European Road Safety Action Programme. Halving the number of road accident victims in the European Union by 2010: a shared responsibility.* Brussels, Commission of the European Communities, 2003 (Com(2003) 311 final)(http://europa.eu.int/comm/transport/road/roadsafety/rsap/index_en.htm, accessed 17 November 2003).

88. O'Neill B, Mohan D. Reducing motor vehicle crash deaths and injuries in newly motorising countries. *British Medical Journal*, 2002, 324:1142–1145.

89. *Road safety committee inquiry into road safety for older road users.* Melbourne, Parliament of Victoria, 2003 (Parliamentary Paper No, 41, Session 2003).

90. Pritz HB. *Effects of hood and fender design on pedestrian head protection.* Washington, DC, National Highway Traffic Safety Administration, 1984 (NHTSA Report No. DOT HS-806-537).

91. Bly PH. Vehicle engineering to protect vulnerable road users. *Journal of Traffic Medicine*, 1990, 18:244.

92. *Proposals for methods to evaluate pedestrian protection for passenger cars.* European Enhanced Vehicle-safety Committee, EEVC Working Group 10, 1994.

93. Crandall JR, Bhalla KS, Madely J. Designing road vehicles for pedestrian protection. *British Medical Journal*, 2002, 324:1145–1148.

94. Hobbs A. *Safer car fronts for pedestrians and cyclists.* Brussels, European Transport Safety Council, 2001 (http://www.etsc.be/pre_06feb01.pdf, accessed 9 December 2003).

95. *Improved test methods to evaluate pedestrian protection afforded by passenger cars.* European Enhanced Vehicle-safety Committee, EEVC Working Group 17, 1998 (http://www.eevc.org/publicdocs/WG17_Improved_test_methods_updated_sept_2002.pdf, accessed 4 December 2003).

96. *Tomorrow's roads: safer for everyone.* London, Department of Environment, Transport and the Regions, 2000.

97. Lawrence GJL, Hardy BJ, Donaldson WMS. *Costs and benefits of the Honda Civic's pedestrian protection, and benefits of the EEVC and ACEA test proposals.* Crowthorne, Transport Research Laboratory, 2002 (Unpublished Project Report PR SE/445/02).

98. Allsop R. *Road safety: Britain in Europe.* London, Parliamentary Advisory Council for Transport Safety, 2001 (http://www.pacts.org.uk/richardslecture.htm, accessed 30 October 2003).

99. *Preliminary report on the development of a global technical regulation concerning pedestrian safety.* United Nations Economic Commission for Europe, 2003 (Trans/WP.29/2003/99, 26 August 2003) (http://www.unece.org/trans/main/welcwp29.htm, accessed 22 December 2003).

100. Roberts I, Mohan D, Abbasi K. War on the roads. *British Medical Journal*, 2002, 324:1107–1108.

101. Chawla A et al. Safer truck front design for pedestrian impacts. *Journal of Crash Prevention and Injury Control*, 2000, 2:33–43.

102. Kajzer J, Yang JK, Mohan D. Safer bus fronts for pedestrian impact protection in bus-pedestrian accidents. In: *Proceedings of the International Research Council on the Biomechanics of Impact (IRCOBI) Conference, Verona, Italy, 9–11 September 1992*. Bron, International Research Council on the Biomechanics of Impact, 1992:13–23.

103. *What is frontal offset crash testing?* Arlington, VA, Insurance Institute for Highway Safety/Highway Loss Data Institute, 2003 (http://www.iihs.org/vehicle_ratings/ce/offset.htm, accessed 10 December 2003).

104. Edwards MJ et al. Review of the frontal and side impact directives. In: *Vehicle Safety 2000, Institute of Mechanical Engineers Conference, London, 7–9 June 2000*. London, Professional Engineering Publishing Limited, 2000.

105. Parkin S, Mackay GM, Frampton RJ. Effectiveness and limitations of current seat belts in Europe. *Chronic Diseases in Canada*, 1992, 14: 38–46.

106. Cummings P et al. Association of driver air bags with driver fatality: a matched cohort study. *British Medical Journal*, 2002, 324:1119–1122.

107. Ferguson SA, Lund AK, Greene MA. *Driver fatalities in 1985–94 airbag cars*. Arlington, VA, Insurance Institute for Highway Safety/Highway Loss Data Institute, 1995.

108. *Fifth/sixth report to Congress: effectiveness of occupant protection systems and their use*. Washington, DC, National Highway Traffic Safety Administration, 2001 (DOT-HS-809-442) (http://www-nrd.nhtsa.dot.gov/pdf/nrd-30/NCSA/Rpts/2002/809-442.pdf, accessed 10 December 2003).

109. *Collision and consequence*. Borlänge, Swedish National Road Administration, 2003 (http://www.vv.se/for_lang/english/publications/C&C.pdf, accessed 10 December 2003).

110. *Initiatives to address vehicle compatibility*. Washington, DC, National Highway Traffic Safety Administration, 2003 (http://www-nrd.nhtsa.dot.gov/departments/nrd-11/aggressivity/IPTVehicleCompatibilityReport/, accessed 22 December 2003).

111. Knight I. *A review of fatal accidents involving agricultural vehicles or other commercial vehicles not classified as a goods vehicle, 1993 to 1995*. Crowthorne, Transport Research Laboratory, 2001 (TRL Report No. 498).

112. Schoon CC. *Invloed kwaliteit fiets op ongevallen [The influence of cycle quality on crashes]*. Leidschendam, Institute for Road Safety Research, 1996 (SWOV Report R-96-32).

113. *Road safety: impact of new technologies*. Paris, Organisation for Economic Co-operation and Development, 2003.

114. *Intelligent transportation systems and road safety*. Brussels, European Transport Safety Council, Working Party of Road Transport Telematics, 1999 (http://www.etsc.be/systems.pdf, accessed 10 December 2003).

115. Westefeld A, Phillips BM. *Effectiveness of various safety belt warning systems*. Washington, DC, National Highway Traffic Safety Administration, 1976 (DOT-HS-801-953).

116. Lie A, Tingvall C. Governmental status report, Sweden. In: *Proceedings of the 18th Experimental Safety of Vehicles Conference, Nagoya, Japan, 19–22 May 2003*. Washington, DC, National Highway Traffic Safety Administration, 2003 (http://www-nrd.nhtsa.dot.gov/pdf/nrd-01/esv/esv18/CD/Files/18ESV-000571.pdf, accessed 10 December 2003).

117. Larsson J, Nilsson, G. *Bältespåminnare: en lönsam trafiksäkerhetsåtgärd? [Seat-belt reminders: beneficial for society?]*. Linköping, Swedish National Road and Transport Research Institute, 2000 (VTI Report 62-2000).

118. Williams AF, Wells JK, Farmer CM. Effectiveness of Ford's belt reminder system in increasing seat belt use. *Injury Prevention*, 2002, 8: 293–296.

119. Williams AF, Wells JK. Drivers' assessment of Ford's belt reminder system. *Traffic Injury Prevention*, 2003, 4:358–362.

120. *Buckling up technologies to increase seat belt use*. Washington, DC, Committee for the Safety Belt Technology Study, The National Academies, in press (Special Report 278).

121. Fildes B et al. *Benefits of seat belt reminder systems*. Canberra, Australian Transport Safety Bureau, 2003 (Report CR 211).

122. Carsten O, Fowkes M, Tate F. *Implementing intelligent speed adaptation in the United Kingdom: recommendations*

of the EVSC project. Leeds, Institute of Transport Studies, University of Leeds, 2001.

123. Marques PR et al. Support services provided during interlock usage and post-interlock repeat DUI: outcomes and processes. In: Laurell H, Schlyter F, eds. *Proceedings of the 15th International Conference on Alcohol, Drugs and Traffic Safety, Stockholm, 22–26 May 2000.* Stockholm, Swedish National Road Administration, 2000 (http://www.vv.se/traf_sak/t2000/908.pdf, accessed 12 December 2003).

124. ICADTS working group on alcohol interlocks. *Alcohol ignition interlock devices. I: Position paper.* Ottawa, International Council on Alcohol, Drugs and Traffic Safety, 2001 (http://www.icadts.org/reports/AlcoholInterlockReport.pdf, accessed 17 December 2003).

125. Tingvall C et al. The effectiveness of ESP (electronic stability programme) in reducing real life accidents. In: *Proceedings of the 18th Experimental Safety of Vehicles Conference, Nagoya, Japan, 19–22 May 2003.* Washington, DC, National Highway Traffic Safety Administration, 2003 (http://www-nrd.nhtsa.dot.gov/pdf/nrd-01/esv/esv18/CD/Files/18ESV-000261.pdf, accessed 12 December 2003).

126. Zaal D. *Traffic law enforcement: a review of the literature.* Melbourne, Monash University Accident Research Centre, 1994 (Report No. 53) (http://www.general.monash.edu.au/muarc/rptsum/muarc53.pdf, accessed 12 December 2003).

127. Redelmeier DA, Tibshirani RJ, Evans L. Traffic-law enforcement and risk of death from motor-vehicle crashes: case-crossover study. *Lancet,* 2003, 361:2177–2182.

128. *Police enforcement strategies to reduce traffic casualties in Europe.* Brussels, European Transport Safety Council, Working Party on Traffic Regulation Enforcement, 1999 (http://www.etsc.be/strategies.pdf, accessed 12 December 2003).

129. Finch DJ et al. *Speed, speed limits and accidents.* Crowthorne, Transport Research Laboratory Ltd, 1994 (Project Report 58).

130. *Reducing injuries from excess and inappropriate speed.* Brussels, European Transport Safety Council, Working Party on Road Infrastructure, 1995.

131. Leggett LMW. The effect on accident occurrence of long-term, low-intensity police enforcement. In: *Proceedings of the 14th Conference of the Australian Road Research Board, Canberra.* Canberra, Australian Road Research Board, 1988, 14:92–104.

132. Keall MD, Povey LJ, Frith WJ. The relative effectiveness of a hidden versus a visible speed camera programme. *Accident Analysis and Prevention,* 2001, 33:277–284.

133. Yang BM, Kim J. Road traffic accidents and policy interventions in Korea. *Injury Control and Safety Promotion,* 2003, 10:89–94.

134. Gains A et al. *A cost recovery system for speed and red light cameras: two year pilot evaluation.* London, Department for Transport, 2003 (http://www.dft.gov.uk/stellent/groups/dft_rdsafety/documents/page/dft_rdsafety_507639.pdf, accessed 12 December 2003) .

135. Mäkinen T, Oei HL. *Automatic enforcement of speed and red light violations: applications, experiences and developments.* Leidschendam, Institute for Road Safety Research, 1992 (Report R-92-58).

136. Brekke G. Automatisk trafikkontroll: har spart Bergen for 40 personskadeulykker [Automatic traffic control: 40 cases of bodily injury averted in Bergen]. In: *Veg i Vest [Roads in Western Norway].* Bergen, Norwegian National Road Authority, 1993, 3:6–7.

137. Elvik R, Mysen AB, Vaa T. *Trafikksikkerhetshåndbok,* tredje utgave *[Handbook of traffic safety, 3rd ed].* Oslo, Institute of Transport Economics, 1997.

138. Mann RE et al. The effects of introducing or lowering legal per se blood alcohol limits for driving: an international review. *Accident Analysis and Prevention,* 2001, 33:569–583.

139. Compton RP et al. Crash risk of alcohol impaired driving. In: Mayhew DR, Dussault C, eds. *Proceedings of the 16th International Conference on Alcohol, Drugs and Traffic Safety, Montreal, 4–9 August 2002.* Montreal, Société de l'assurance automobile du Québec, 2002:39–44 (http://www.saaq.gouv.qc.ca/t2002/actes/pdf/(06a).pdf, accessed 17 November 2003).

140. Stewart K et al. International comparisons of laws and alcohol crash rates: lessons learned. In: Laurell H, Schlyter F, eds. *Proceedings of the 15th International Conference on Alcohol, Drugs and Traffic Safety,*

Stockholm, 22–26 May 2000, Stockholm, Swedish National Road Administration, 2000 (http://www.vv.se/traf_sak/t2000/541.pdf, accessed 17 November 2003).

141. Davis A et al. *Improving road safety by reducing impaired driving in LMICs: a scoping study.* Crowthorne, Transport Research Laboratory, 2003 (Project Report 724/03).

142. Assum T. *Road safety in Africa: appraisal of road safety initiatives in five African countries.* Washington, DC, The World Bank and United Nations Economic Commission for Africa, 1998 (Working Paper No. 33).

143. Howat P, Sleet DA, Smith DI. Alcohol and driving: is the 0.05 blood alcohol concentration limit justified? *Drug and Alcohol Review,* 1991, 10:151–166.

144. Jonah B et al. The effects of lowering legal blood alcohol limits for driving: a review. In: Laurell H, Schlyter F, eds. *Proceedings of the 15th International Conference on Alcohol, Drugs and Traffic Safety, Stockholm, 22–26 May 2000.* Stockholm, Swedish National Road Administration, 2000 (http://www.vv.se/traf_sak/t2000/522.pdf, accessed 15 December 2003).

145. Shults RA et al. Reviews of evidence regarding interventions to reduce alcohol-impaired driving. *American Journal of Preventive Medicine,* 2001, 21:66–88.

146. Miller TR, Lestina DC, Spicer RS. Highway crash costs in the United States by driver age, blood alcohol level, victim age and restraint use. *Accident Analysis and Prevention,* 1998, 30:137–150.

147. Sweedler BM. Strategies for dealing with the persistent drinking driver. In: *Proceedings of the 13th International Conference on Alcohol, Drugs and Traffic Safety, Adelaide, 13–18 August 1995.* Adelaide, University of Adelaide, Road Accident Research Unit, 1995 (http://casr.adelaide.edu.au/T95/paper/s1p3.html, accessed 16 December 2003).

148. Homel RJ. Random breath testing in Australia: a complex deterrent. *Australian Drug and Alcohol Review,* 1988, 7:231–241.

149. Elder RW et al. Effectiveness of sobriety checkpoints for reducing alcohol-involved crashes. *Traffic Injury Prevention,* 2002, 3:266–274.

150. Eckhardt A, Seitz E. *Wirtschaftliche Bewertung von Sicherheitsmassnahmen [Economic elaboration of safety measures].* Berne, Swiss Council for Accident Prevention, 1998 (Report No. 35).

151. Arthurson RM. *Evaluation of random breath testing.* Sydney, New South Wales Traffic Authority, 1985 (Report RN 10/85).

152. Camkin HL, Webster KA. *Cost-effectiveness and priority ranking of road safety measures.* Roseberry, New South Wales Traffic Authority, 1988 (Report RN 1/88).

153. Stuster JW, Blowers PA. *Experimental evaluation of sobriety checkpoint programs.* Washington, DC, National Highway Traffic Safety Administration, 1995 (DOT HS-808-287).

154. Miller TR, Galbraith MS, Lawrence BA. Costs and benefits of a community sobriety checkpoint program. *Journal of Studies on Alcohol,* 1998, 59:462–468.

155. Elder RW et al. Effectiveness of mass media campaigns for reducing drinking and driving and alcohol-involved crashes: a systematic review. *American Journal of Preventive Medicine,* in press.

156. Guria J, Leung J. An evaluation of a supplementary road safety package. In: *25th Australasian Transport Research Forum, Canberra, 2–4 October 2002* (http://www.btre.gov.au/docs/atrf_02/papers/36GuriaLeung.doc, accessed 7 January 2004).

157. Ross HL. Punishment as a factor in preventing alcohol-related accidents. *Addiction,* 1993, 88:997–1002.

158. *Reducing injuries from alcohol impairment.* Brussels, European Transport Safety Council, 1995.

159. Wells-Parker E et al. Final results from a meta-analysis of remedial interventions with drink/drive offenders. *Addiction,* 1995, 90:907–926.

160. Maycock G. *Driver sleepiness as a factor in cars and HGV accidents.* Crowthorne, Transport Research Laboratory Ltd, 1995 (Report No. 169).

161. *The role of driver fatigue in commercial road transport crashes.* Brussels, European Transport Safety Council, 2001 (http://www.etsc.be/drivfatigue.pdf, accessed 15 December 2003).

162. *Drowsy driving and automobile crashes: report and recommendations.* Washington, DC, National Center on Sleep Disorder Research and National Highway Traffic Safety Administration, Expert Panel

on Driver Fatigue and Sleepiness, 1996 (http://www.nhlbi.nih.gov/health/prof/sleep/drsy_drv.pdf, accessed 15 December 2003).

163. Hartley LR et al. *Comprehensive review of fatigue research*. Fremantle, Murdoch University, Institute for Research in Safety and Transport, 1996 (http://www.psychology.murdoch.edu.au/irst/publ/Comprehensive_Review_of_Fatigue_Research.pdf, accessed 15 December 2003).

164. Mock C, Amegeshi J, Darteh K. Role of commercial drivers in motor vehicle related injuries in Ghana. *Injury Prevention*, 1999, 5:268–271.

165. Nantulya VM, Muli-Musiime F. Uncovering the social determinants of road traffic accidents in Kenya. In: Evans T et al., eds. *Challenging inequities: from ethics to action*. Oxford, Oxford University Press, 2001:211–225.

166. Nafukho FM, Khayesi M. Livelihood, conditions of work, regulation and road safety in the small-scale public transport sector: a case of the *Matatu* mode of transport in Kenya. In: Godard X, Fatonzoun I, eds. *Urban mobility for all. Proceedings of the Tenth International CODATU Conference, Lome, Togo, 12–15 November 2002*. Lisse, AA Balkema Publishers, 2002:241–245.

167. Morris JR. External accident costs and freight transport efficiency. In: Saccomanno F, Shortreed J, eds. *Truck safety: perceptions and reality*. Waterloo, Institute for Risk Research, 1996.

168. Hamelin P. Lorry drivers' time habits in work and their involvement in traffic accidents. *Ergonomics*, 1987, 30:1323–1333.

169. South DR et al. *Evaluation of the red light camera programme and the owner onus legislation*. Melbourne, Traffic Authority, 1988.

170. Red light cameras yield big reductions in crashes and injuries. *Status Report*, 2001, 36:1–8.

171. Hooke A, Knox J, Portas D. *Cost benefit analysis of traffic light and speed cameras*. London, Home Office, Police Research Group, 1996 (Police Research Series Paper 20).

172. *Seat-belts and child restraints: increasing use and optimising performance*. Brussels, European Transport Safety Council, 1996.

173. Heiman L. *Vehicle occupant protection in Australia*. Canberra, Australian Transport Safety Bureau, 1988.

174. Ashton SJ, Mackay GM, Camm S. Seat belt use in Britain under voluntary and mandatory conditions. In: *Proceedings of the 27th Conference of the American Association for Automotive Medicine (AAAM)*. Chicago, IL, American Association for Automotive Medicine, 1983:65–75.

175. Rutherford W et al. *The medical effects of seat belt legislation in the United Kingdom*. London, Department of Health and Social Security, Office of the Chief Scientist, 1985 (Research Report No. 13).

176. Rivara FP et al. Systematic reviews of strategies to prevent motor vehicle injuries. *American Journal of Preventive Medicine*, 1999, 16:1–5.

177. Dinh-Zarr et al. Reviews of evidence regarding interventions to increase the use of safety belts. *American Journal of Preventive Medicine*, 2001, 21:48–65.

178. Shults R et al. Primary enforcement seat belt laws are effective even in the face of rising belt use rates. *Accident Analysis and Prevention*, in press.

179. Jonah BA, Dawson NE, Smith GA. Effects of a selective traffic enforcement program on seat belt use. *Journal of Applied Psychology*, 1982, 67:89–96.

180. Jonah BA, Grant BA. Long-term effectiveness of selective traffic enforcement programs for increasing seat belt use. *Journal of Applied Psychology*, 1985, 70:257–263.

181. Gundy C. The effectiveness of a combination of police enforcement and public information for improving seat belt use. In: Rothengatter JA, de Bruin RA, eds. *Road user behaviour: theory and research*. Assen, Van Gorcum, 1988.

182. Solomon MG, Ulmer RG, Preusser DF. *Evaluation of click it or ticket model programs*. Washington, DC, National Highway Traffic Safety Administration, 2002 (DOT HS-809-498).

183. Solomon MG, Chaudhary NK, Cosgrove LA. *Evaluation of the May 2003 mobilization: programs to increase safety belt usage*. Washington, DC, National Highway Traffic Safety Administration, in press.

184. Hagenzieker M. Effects of incentives on safety belt use: a meta-analysis. *Crash Analysis and Prevention*, 1997, 29:759–777.

185. Koch D, Medgyesi M, Landry P. *Saskatchewan's occupant restraint program (1988–94): performance to date*. Regina, Saskatchewan Government Insurance, 1995.

186. Dussault C. Effectiveness of a selective traffic enforcement program combined with incentives for seat belt use in Quebec. *Health Education Research: Theory and Practice*, 1990, 5:217–223.

187. Aekplakorn W et al. Compliance with the law on car seat-belt use in four cities of Thailand. *Journal of the Medical Association of Thailand*, 2000, 83:333–341.

188. Morrison DS, Petticrew M, Thomson H. What are the most effective ways of improving population health through transport interventions? Evidence from systematic reviews. *Journal of Epidemiology and Community Health*, 2003, 57: 327–333.

189. *Carrying children safely.* Birmingham, Royal Society for the Prevention of Accidents, 2002 (http://www.childcarseats.org.uk/factsheets/carrying_safely_factsheet.pdf, accessed 16 December 2003).

190. Zaza S et al. Reviews of evidence regarding interventions to increase use of child safety seats. *American Journal of Preventive Medicine*, 2001, 21:31–43.

191. Motor vehicle occupant injury: strategies for increasing use of child safety seats, increasing use of safety belts and reducing alcohol-impaired driving. A report on recommendations of the task force on community preventive services. *Mobility and Mortality Weekly Report*, 2001, 50:7 (http://www.cdc.gov/mmwr/PDF/RR/RR5007.pdf, accessed 16 December 2003).

192. Mohan D, Schneider L. An evaluation of adult clasping strength for restraining lap held infants. *Human Factors*, 1979, 21:635–645.

193. Anund A et al. *Child safety in care: literature review.* Linköping, Swedish National Road and Transport Research Institute, 2003 (VTI Report 489A9)(http://www.vti.se/PDF/reports/R489A.pdf, accessed 7 December 2003).

194. Thompson DC, Rivara FP, Thompson RS. Effectiveness of bicycle helmets in preventing head injuries: a case-control study. *Journal of the American Medical Association*, 1996, 276:1968–1973.

195. Thompson DC, Rivara FP, Thompson R. Helmets for preventing head and facial injuries in bicyclists. *Cochrane Database of Systematic Reviews*, 2000, (2):CD001855.

196. Sosin DM, Sacks JJ, Webb KW. Pediatric head injuries and deaths from bicycling in the United States. *Pediatrics*, 1996, 98:868–870.

197. Towner E et al. *Bicycle helmets – a review of their effectiveness: a critical review of the literature.* London, Department of Transport, 2002 (Road Safety Research Report No. 30).

198. LeBlanc JC, Beattie TL, Culligan C. Effect of legislation on the use of bicycle helmets. *Canadian Medical Association Journal*, 2002, 166:592–595.

199. Coffman S. Bicycle injuries and safety helmets in children: review of research. *Orthopaedic Nursing*, 2003, 22:9–15.

200. Thompson RS, Rivara FP, Thompson DC. A case-control study of the effectiveness of bicycle safety helmets. *New England Journal of Medicine*, 1989, 320:1361–1367.

201. Attewell RG, Glase K, McFadden M. Bicycle helmet efficacy: a meta analysis. *Accident Analysis and Prevention*, 2001, 33:345–352.

202. Macpherson AK et al. Impact of mandatory helmet legislation on bicycle-related head injuries in children: a population-based study. *Pediatrics*, 2002, 110:e60.

203. Scuffham P et al. Head injuries to bicyclists and the New Zealand bicycle helmet law. *Accident Analysis and Prevention*, 2000, 32:565–573.

204. Macpherson AK, Macarthur C. Bicycle helmet legislation: evidence for effectiveness. *Pediatric Research*, 2002, 52:472.

205. Vulcan P, Cameron MH, Watson WC. Mandatory bicycle helmet use: experience in Victoria, Australia. *World Journal of Surgery*, 1992, 16:389–397.

206. Povey LJ, Frith WJ, Graham PG. Cycle helmet effectiveness in New Zealand. *Accident Analysis and Prevention*, 1999, 31:763–770.

207. Graitcer P, Kellerman A, Christoffel T. A review of educational and legislative strategies to promote bicycle helmets. *Injury Prevention*, 1995, 1:122–129.

208. Liller KD et al. Children's bicycle helmet use and injuries in Hillsborough County, Florida, before and after helmet legislation. *Injury Prevention*, 2003, 9:177–179.

209. *Motorcycle safety helmets. COST 327.* Brussels, Commission of the European Communities, 2001 (http://www.cordis.lu/cost-transport/src/cost-327.htm, accessed 17 November 2003).

210.Radin Umar RS. Helmet initiatives in Malaysia. In: *Proceedings of the 2nd World Engineering Congress.* Sarawak, Institution of Engineers, 2002: 93–101.

211. Supramaniam V, Belle V, Sung J. Fatal motorcycle accidents and helmet laws in Peninsular Malaysia. *Accident Analysis and Prevention*, 1984, 16: 157–162.

212.Ichikawa M, Chadbunchachai W, Marui E. Effect of the helmet act for motorcyclists in Thailand. *Accident Analysis and Prevention*, 2003, 35: 183–189.

213.Servadei F et al. Effects of Italy's motorcycle helmet law on traumatic brain injuries. *Injury Prevention*, 2003, 9:257–260.

214.Ulmer RG, Preusser DF. *Evaluation of the repeal of the motorcycle helmet laws in Kentucky and Louisiana.* Washington, DC, National Highway Traffic Safety Administration, 2003 (Report No. DOT HS-809-530).

215.Waters H, Hyder AA, Phillips T. Economic evaluation of interventions to reduce road traffic injuries: a review of the literature with applications to low and middle income countries. *Asia Pacific Journal of Public Health*, in press.

216.Johnston I. Traffic safety education: panacea, prophylactic or placebo? *World Journal of Surgery*, 1992, 16:374–376.

217. O'Neill B et al. The World Bank's Global Road Safety and Partnership. *Traffic Injury Prevention*, 2002, 3:190–194.

218.Duperrex O, Bunn F, Roberts I. Safety education of pedestrians for injury prevention: a systematic review of randomised controlled trials. *British Medical Journal*, 2002, 324:1129.

219. Ker K et al. Post-licence driver education for the prevention of road traffic crashes. *Cochrane Database of Systematic Reviews*, 2003, (3):CD003734.

220.Dueker RL. *Experimental field test of proposed anti-dart-out training programs. Volume 1. Conduct and results.* Valencia, PA, Applied Science Associates Inc, 1981.

221.Ytterstad B. The Harstad injury prevention study: hospital-based injury recording used for outcome evaluation of community-based prevention of bicyclist and pedestrian injury.

Scandinavian Journal of Primary Health Care, 1995, 13: 141–149.

222.Schioldborg P. Children, traffic and traffic training: analysis of the Children's Traffic Club. *The Voice of the Pedestrian*, 1976, 6:12–19.

223.Bryan-Brown K. The effects of a children's traffic club. In: *Road accidents: Great Britain 1994. The Casualty Report.* London, Her Majesty's Stationery Office, 1995:55–61.

224.Blomberg RD et al. *Experimental field test of proposed pedestrian safety messages. Volume I: Methods and materials development.* Washington, DC, National Highway Traffic Safety Administration, 1983 (DOT-HS-4-00952).

225.*Reducing the severity of road injuries through post impact care.* Brussels, European Transport Safety Council, Post Impact Care Working Party, 1999.

226.Lerner EB, Moscati RM. The golden hour: scientific fact or medical "urban legend". *Academic Emergency Medicine*, 2001, 8:758–760.

227.Mock CN et al. Trauma mortality patterns in three nations at different economic levels: implications for global trauma system development. *Journal of Trauma*, 1998, 44:804–814.

228.Pang TY et al. *Injury characteristics of Malaysian motorcyclists by Abbreviated Injury Scale (AIS).* Kuala Serdang, Malaysia, Road Safety Research Centre, Universiti Putra Malaysia, 2000 (Research Report RR2/2000).

229.Mock CN, Arreola-Risa C, Quansah R. Strengthening care for injured persons in less developed countries: a case study of Ghana and Mexico. *Injury Control and Safety Promotion*, 2003, 10:45–51.

230.Hussain IM, Redmond AD. Are pre-hospital deaths from accidental injury preventable? *British Medical Journal*, 1994, 308:1077–1080.

231.Forjouh S et al. Transport of the injured to hospitals in Ghana: the need to strengthen the practice of trauma care. *Pre-hospital Immediate Care*, 1999, 3:66–70.

232.Husum H et al. Rural pre-hospital trauma systems improve trauma outcome in low-income countries: a prospective study from north Iraq and Cambodia. *Journal of Trauma*, 2003, 54: 1188–1196.

233. Hauswald M, Yeoh E. Designing a pre-hospital system for a developing country: estimated costs and benefits. *American Journal of Emergency Medicine*, 1997; 15:600–603.

234. Van Rooyen MJ, Thomas TL, Clem KJ. International Emergency Medical Services: assessment of developing prehospital systems abroad. *Journal of Emergency Medical Services*, 1999, 17:691–696.

235. Bunn F et al. *Effectiveness of pre-hospital care: a report by the Cochrane Injuries Group for the World Health Organisation*. London, The Cochrane Injuries Group, 2001.

236. Mock CN, Quansah RE, Addae-Mensah L. Kwame Nkrumah University of Science and Technology continuing medical education course in trauma management. *Trauma Quarterly*, 1999, 14:345–348.

237. *Resources for the optimal care of the injured patient, 1999*. Chicago, IL, American College of Surgeons, Committee on Trauma, 1999.

238. Knight P, Trinca G. The development, philosophy and transfer of trauma care programs. In: *Reflections on the transfer of traffic safety knowledge to motorising nations*. Melbourne, Global Traffic Safety Trust, 1998:75–78.

239. Ali J et al. Trauma outcome improves following the advanced trauma life support program in a developing country. *Journal of Trauma*, 1993, 34: 898–899.

240. Goosen J et al. Trauma care systems in South Africa. *Injury*, 2003, 34:704–708.

241. Quansah R. Availability of emergency medical services along major highways. *Ghana Medical Journal*, 2001, 35:8–10.

242. Nantulya V, Reich M. The neglected epidemic: road traffic injuries in developing countries. *British Medical Journal*, 2002, 324:1139–1141.

243. Mock C et al. *Report on the consultation meeting to develop an essential trauma care programme*. Geneva, World Health Organization, 2002 (WHO/NMH/VIP02.09).

244. Hyder AA. Health research investments: a challenge for national public health associations. *Journal of the Pakistan Medical Association*, 2002, 52:276–277.

245. Hyder AA, Akhter T, Qayyum A. Capacity development for health research in Pakistan: the effect of doctoral training. *Health Policy and Planning*, 2003, 18:338–343.